Orthopaedic Trauma:

A Systematic Approach

Contents

The lower limb

Section 3: Practical procedures

List of contributors

Hesham Al-Khateeb is Specialist Registrar in Trauma and Orthopaedics, London

Thomas Carlstedt is Professor at the Peripheral Nerve Injury Unit, Royal National Orthopaedic Hospital, Stanmore, Middlesex

Brian Cohen is Consultant Orthopaedic Surgeon, The Princess Grace Hospital, London

Aklbar De Medici is Clinical Fellow in Trauma and Orthopaedics, University College Hospitals NHS Trust, London

Fares Haddad is Clinical Director and Orthopaedic Consultant at University College London Hospitals NHS Trust, London

A Reza Jenabzadeh is Specialist Registrar in Trauma and Orthopaedics, London

Daren Forward is Specialist Registrar in Trauma and Orthopaedics at Nottingham University Hospitals NHS Trust, Nottingham

Max Horwitz is Specialist Registrar in Trauma and Orthopaedics, London

Benjamin Hudson is Senior House Officer in the Accident and Emergency Department, University College Hospitals NHS Trust, London

Simon Jennings is Consultant Orthopaedic Surgeon, Northwick Park Hospital, Harrow, Middlesex

Ken Mannan is Specialist Registrar in Trauma and Orthopaedics, London

Christopher Moran is Professor and Consultant Orthopaedic Surgeon, Quenns Medical Centre, Nottingham

Sam Oussedik is Specialist Registrar in Trauma and Orthopaedics, London

Rahul Patel is Specialist Registrar in Trauma and Orthopaedics, London

Elliot D Sorene is Consultant Orthopaedic and Hand Surgeon, University College London Hospitals NHS Trust, London

James Waller is Senior House Officer in the Department of Medicine, Royal Bournemouth Hospital, Bournemouth

Nicholas Wardle is Specialist Registrar in Trauma and Orthopaedics, London

Alexander Woolard is Senior House Officer in Surgery, University College Hospitals NHS Trust, London

Claire Young is Locum Consultant, Darlington NHS Trust, Co Durham

Foreword

This book is intended to cover the basics of the management of common orthopaedic and musculoskeletal injuries for medical students, junior doctors and paramedical staff. The book has been kept at a basic and practical level in order to aid those involved in the initial assessment and management of these patients, to enable them to make the fundamental and critical decisions necessary in a primary and secondary setting and to perform the interventions that are required with appropriate guidance.

This book cannot be comprehensive and exhaustive in terms of orthopaedic trauma nor is it designed to be a bible of accident and emergency surgery. It is a concise summary of basic orthopaedic facts, of common presentations and of injuries and procedures that need to be in the armamentarium of the junior doctor.

The impetus for this book has been the change in medical training with the arrival of modernising medical careers and the foundation curriculum. The editors felt that it was important to outline a series of orthopaedic/musculoskeletal/trauma competencies in a simple, easily digested way for medical students, junior doctors and paramedics.

This project is specifically aimed at juniors. To that end each chapter has been written by a junior doctor who has recently been exposed to the stresses, traumas and difficulties that medical students and junior doctors face but in each case the chapter has been supervised by a more senior colleague with expertise in the subject. Many of the chapters have been modified from a series that was first published in the *British Journal of Hospital Medicine* and the book will of course not have been possible without the foresight of Rebecca Linssen and her colleagues who saw the potential for these topics to be included in both the foundation supplement of *Hospital Medicine* and also amalgamated into this tome. At a practical level, Helena Raeside and Maria Anguita have provided invaluable assistance.

In every project there are a number of significant contributors. I personally owe a massive debt to Sam Oussedik and Rahul Patel. They were involved right at the outset with the development of this idea. They have undertaken primary editing for most of the chapters and have been tireless workers and good friends throughout the process. There are times when they have undoubtedly become tired of my nagging emails yet they have never failed to deliver excellent quality material on time and with good humour.

This book is designed to introduce the reader to basic trauma management and to whet the appetite for further study. It is hoped that it will help you and your patients.

Fares Haddad

Introduction

Trauma is a leading cause of morbidity and mortality in the developed world. Once an individual has been injured, it falls to the medical professionals to firstly preserve life and secondly, and perhaps just as importantly, preserve function. Often a patient's first contact with a medical professional following an injury will be in the accident and emergency department. It is at this juncture that rapid and accurate assessment and initiation of appropriate treatment will ensure an optimal outcome is achieved.

The following chapters have been written with health care professionals in mind. They seek to provide the basic scientific and clinical information necessary to the clinician in providing excellent trauma care. The chapters have been drawn up along anatomical lines and the structure is such that having studied each chapter readers should be able to:

- Understand the significance of injuries to the region.
- Know the clinically relevant anatomy of the region.
- Recognise the common mechanisms of injury.
- Understand how patients commonly present.
- Be able to assess injuries.
- Understand the classification of injuries.
- Recognise which patients require referral to a trauma surgeon.
- Know what can be done in the accident and emergency department to treat each injury.
- Have an insight into how the trauma surgeon might treat the injury.

In this way it is hoped that readers, particularly those encountering trauma cases for the first time, will feel better equipped to accurately assess injured patients and provide initial treatment. Readers should also feel more confident in discussing cases with their senior colleagues and trauma surgeons, improving the referral process.

Each of the chapters could have been written with the same introductory paragraph outlining the initial assessment and treatment of the injured patient. For the sake of brevity this has not been included. It should be stressed that initial treatment steps in all cases should follow the guidelines provided by the Advanced Trauma and Life Support framework. Thus regional trauma is only assessed once the patient has been adequately resuscitated and stabilised.

The first section outlines the principles of trauma care, dealing with adult and paediatric trauma, and discussing the approach to open fractures. These chapters are meant as a brief introduction to the topics and should also point the reader towards other sources of information.

The second section deals with regional trauma. This should provide enough information to allow the reader to feel well informed on each injury. It is not meant as an exhaustive discussion of trauma surgery, and so examples of definitive care are provided to inform the uninitiated rather than guide the expert.

The third section gives guidance in carrying out those practical procedures which are commonly encountered in the accident and emergency department. These should provide a starting point and framework for gaining practical experience. Such procedures are best taught in the clinical setting by senior colleagues, but it is hoped that gaining a little knowledge prior to this should speed the learning process and perhaps make it less painful for patient and clinician alike.

Finally, this book is meant as a reference guide, to be dipped into when required rather than read in one sitting. It is hoped that it will become a valuable resource for all emergency clinicians and perhaps ease the transition from medical student to specialist trainee.

Sam Oussedik

Section One:

Systematic approach to trauma

CHAPTER 1

Principles of adult trauma care

Sam Oussedik and Fares Haddad

Introduction

Polytraumatised patients represent a significant challenge to the emergency department team. Preserving life and function in such patients can be daunting to the uninitiated. The application of a systematic approach to both assessment and treatment provides the clinician with a framework within which to operate, allowing injuries to be diagnosed and treated with optimal efficiency. The guidelines set out by the Advanced Trauma and Life Support (ATLS) programme of the American College of Surgeons (1997) provide such a framework, and completion of an ATLS course is strongly recommended to all healthcare professionals encountering trauma patients on a regular basis.

The trauma team

The majority of emergency departments will have access to a designated trauma team. The make-up of this team may vary from hospital to hospital, but usually includes, in addition to the emergency department clinician:

- Anaesthetist – assesses airway and ventilation and provides support when necessary.
- General surgeon – assesses the abdomen for signs of haemorrhage, hollow viscous or solid organ damage; may also assess urinary tract injuries.
- Trauma surgeon – assesses pelvic and long bone injuries; may also carry out secondary survey.
- Nursing staff – support; intravenous fluids.
- Support staff – radiographer, laboratory staff.

The trauma team may be lead by any of the above staff, this task usually falling to the clinician most experienced in trauma care. The actual make up of the team is less important than the adherence to the principles of trauma care.

Initial patient assessment

Traumatised patients present to the emergency department in a number of

Table 1.1. The Revised Trauma Score

	Variables	Score
A: Respiratory rate (Breaths/min)	10–29	4
	>29	3
	6–9	2
	1–5	1
	0	0
B: Systolic blood pressure (mmHg)	>89	4
	76–89	3
	50–75	2
	1–49	1
	0	0
C: Glasgow Coma Scale	13–15	4
	9–12	3
	6–8	2
	4–5	1
	<4	0

Revised Trauma Score = A + B + C (Champion *et al*, 1989).
While the Revised Trauma Score has been shown to be a poor predictor of outcome, it does act as a useful triage tool to ensure variables are measured

different ways. Whether brought in by ambulance or self-presenting, a rapid and reliable way of triaging patients is necessary. This is usually carried out by the first healthcare provider to encounter the patient, be this the ambulance crew or the specially trained emergency department nursing staff, who will assess:

- Vital signs – blood pressure, heart rate, respiratory rate, conscious level (Revised Trauma Score – *Table 1.1*).
- Injury pattern – head injury, chest injury, abdominal injury, long bone fracture.
- Injury energy – high speed road traffic accident, fall from a height, fall from standing.
- Patient reserve – elderly, pregnant, pre-existing cardiac/respiratory/renal disease, diabetes.

A rapid assessment of which patients might require urgent care can therefore be made.

The primary survey

The next phase of trauma care is the primary survey. This follows a defined sequence:

A: Airway maintenance and cervical spine control
B: Breathing and ventilation
C: Circulation and haemorrhage control
D: Disability
E: Exposure and environmental control

The underlying principle to this assessment is that life-threatening conditions are diagnosed and treated as they are encountered. In the presence of a trauma team it is not unusual for all of the above phases to be carried out simultaneously by different team members. The allocation of roles to team members prior to commencement facilitates this process.

Airway maintenance and cervical spine control

The airway is assessed to ensure patency. In the presence of a speaking patient this can often be a rapid process. However, complications may arise with head and facial injuries or with altered conscious level. A Glasgow Coma Scale (GCS, *Table 1.2*) score of less than 8 is a relative indication to definitive airway placement. It is while assessing the airway and during manoeuvres to protect it that the cervical spine is at its most vulnerable, hence the inclusion of cervical spine control at this early juncture. Cervical spine injury should be suspected in all patients with a history of significant energy trauma, and steps taken to protect the cervical spine until such injuries are ruled out.

Breathing and ventilation

Having ensured airway patency, it is now imperative to ensure adequate ventilation and gas exchange. Oxygen saturations and respiratory rate measurement are useful adjuncts to this process but do not remove the necessity of chest auscultation and examination of excursion. Injuries to the chest wall, diaphragm and/or lungs may impede gas exchange. Life-threatening injuries include tension pneumothorax, massive pneumothorax, open pneumothorax and haemothorax. These should be actively excluded before moving on.

Circulation and haemorrhage control

Tissue oxygenation is dependent on the gases exchanged within the lungs being

Table 1.2. The Glasgow Coma Scale. Scores in the three areas are added to give an overall score out of 15

Eye opening	Spontaneous	4
	To speech	3
	To pain	2
	None	1
Best motor response	Obeys commands	6
	Localises pain	5
	Withdrawal	4
	Flexion	3
	Extension	2
	None	1
Verbal response	Orientated	5
	Confused	4
	Inappropriate	3
	Incomprehensible	2
	None	1

transported to and from the organs. This requires the circulation of a sufficient concentration of haemoglobin at an adequate pressure. The important factors can be summarised in the following manner:

Cardiac output (CO) = stroke volume (SV) x heart rate (HR)
Blood pressure (BP) = CO x systemic vascular resistance (SVR)
Therefore: BP = SV x HR x SVR

In the absence of cardiac injury or a history of significant cardiac disease, cardiac output is therefore dependent on the stroke volume and the heart rate. Stroke volume is in turn dependent on the filling pressure of the left ventricle, while heart rate and systemic vascular resistance in trauma patients is often raised in the presence of a catecholamine response. The single most modifiable value is therefore that of stroke volume, which will in turn control blood pressure. Stroke volume can be increased by preventing external haemorrhage by means of compression, treating internal haemorrhage when encountered by operative means if necessary, and volume repletion by intravenous infusion. Long bone fractures are also sources of haemorrhage, and initial splinting of such injuries can help to reduce the volume lost.

Disability

The patient's response to stimuli is assessed by means of the Glasgow Coma Scale (*Table 1.2*). The patient's pupil reactivity is also assessed.

Conscious level can be impaired in the presence of increased intracranial pressure, alcohol, drugs, hypoxia and hypotension. If these last two factors are excluded then decreased conscious level should be attributed to head injury until proven otherwise.

Exposure and environmental control

The patient is fully exposed such that any potential injuries can be seen. It is important however to ensure that the patient remains warm following this, by the application of warming blankets when necessary.

Having completed the primary survey, the process is then repeated to ensure no deterioration has occurred. Only once life-threatening injuries have been excluded or diagnosed and treated can the secondary survey be carried out.

The secondary survey

This is a top-to-toe examination of the patient, assessing the presence of further, non-life-threatening injuries. A full history may be taken at this point. Skeletal trauma is assessed as set out in the following chapters. Having preserved life during the primary survey, it is now imperative to preserve function by diagnosing and treating all injuries.

Conclusion

Adult trauma care is best undertaken by implementing a systematic approach based on sound anatomical and physiological principles. Treating life-threatening injuries as soon as they are identified before moving on to life-altering injuries represents the best approach. Adherence to these principles allows the clinician to begin gaining the practical experience on which good trauma care is based.

Key points

- Trauma patients are initially triaged to identify those who may be at immediate risk.
- The primary survey follows the approach laid out by the ATLS guidelines, evaluating injuries in the order in which they may prove fatal.
- Life-threatening conditions are diagnosed and treated as they are encountered.
- A secondary survey of non-life-threatening injuries is only carried out once the primary survey and resulting treatment is complete.

References

American College of Surgeons (1997) *Advanced Trauma and Life Support – Student Course Manual* (6th Edn.) American College of Surgeons, Chicago.

Champion HR, Sacco WJ, Copes WS, Gann DS, Gennarelli TA, Flanagan ME (1989) A revision of the Trauma Score. *J Trauma* **29(5)**: 623–9.

CHAPTER 2

Principles of paediatric injuries

A Reza Jenabzadeh and Fares Haddad

Introduction

Trauma is the most common cause of death in children over the age of one year. Mechanisms of injury include non-accidental injury, falls, and road traffic accidents. The ratio of boys to girls is two to one. The peak incidence of fractures in boys occurs at age 16 and in girls at age 12. Paediatric injuries differ from those in adults in many respects. This chapter discusses why this is the case and outlines the general principles of treating paediatric injuries. It will also look at non-accidental injury (NAI), which should always be considered when reviewing a child with a fracture.

Anatomy

Skeletal trauma accounts for 10–15% of all childhood injuries, with approximately 15% of these representing physeal injuries. Fractures in children have some unique characteristics and differences from those in adults. While the injured adult has to recover from the trauma itself, children also need to cope with any effects of the trauma on their growth.

Children's bones have a higher water content and lower mineral content per unit volume than adult bone. Therefore, paediatric bone is more elastic (less brittle) and has a higher strain to failure ratio. As a general rule, ligaments in children are functionally stronger than are bones. Thus, a high proportion of injuries that produce sprains in adults result in fractures in children.

The biomechanical characteristics of the growing skeleton are also different. Children's bones are more malleable, allowing a plastic type of 'bowing' injury. This may lead to an incomplete fracture (greenstick), which occurs more often in children.

Bone healing is faster in children and complications affecting bone healing are rarer than in adults because the bone is more biologically active with a thick vascular periosteum. The thicker periosteum is more highly developed than in adults and usually remains intact on the concave side of the fracture. This helps stabilise any reduction, decreases the amount of displacement, and is probably a factor in the lower incidence of open fractures in children than in adults. Stiffness across joints after immobilisation is less of a problem in children than in adults.

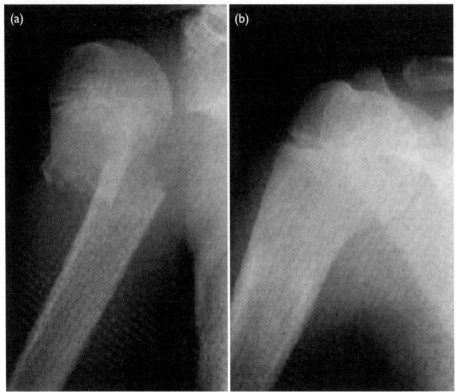

Figure 2.1. (a) Fracture of the proximal humerus at 6 years of age. (b) The same fracture after conservative treatment aged 10 years. The fracture was not treated operatively as doctors knew it would remodel.

Children's bones remodel to a greater extent than do adults (*Figure 2.1*), and therefore a greater amount of angulation and displacement is acceptable in children (apart from intra-articular fractures where angulation or displacement is not acceptable at all). As a general rule, the younger the patient is, the greater the remodelling potential; thus absolute anatomical reduction in a child is less important than in a comparable injury in an adult. However, rotational deformity does not correct so readily in the young child and should be avoided. Apposition and mild shortening are of little importance in young children. Apposition and remodelling is acceptable in boys under the age of 12 years and girls under 10 years of age. Slight shortening with reduction may be desirable in the leg because acceleration of growth occurs after a displaced fracture.

The long bones of children have epiphyses and physes, the latter of which seem to be the weakest point of the child's skeleton, accounting for the difference between the location of fractures in children and adults. The biomechanical properties change with age and there are characteristic injury patterns for different age groups. Fractures involving the physis only occur in

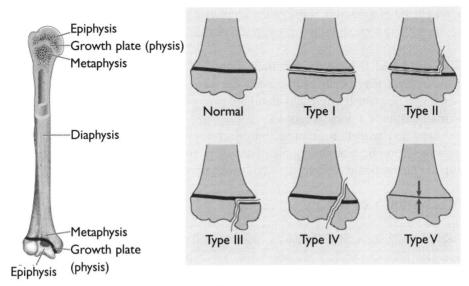

Figure 2.2. *Salter Harris classification of epiphyseal plate injuries I–V.*

children. The physes should be kept in as near normal condition as possible to avoid growth arrest and angular deformities.

Physeal (growth plate) injuries

Physeal injuries are usually caused by torsion (not tension) at the growth plates. The most common sites for physeal arrest are at the distal femur, distal radius, distal tibia and proximal tibia. Complications of physeal injuries include limb length discrepancies, malunions and physeal arrest. Trauma is the commonest cause of physeal arrest. Computed tomography (CT) and magnetic resonance imaging (MRI) are useful for diagnosing a physeal arrest. Arrest occurs when a bridge of bone (physeal bar) forms between the metaphysis and epiphysis. The uninjured portion may continue to grow. Centrally located bars within the physis lead to arrest of longitudinal growth with resultant shortening of the extremity. Peripheral bars (the most common pattern) lead to angular deformities. The magnitude of the resultant deformity is determined by the remaining growth of the child as well as the location of the bar.

Salter and Harris came up with a classification system for physeal fractures (*Figure 2.2*).

- Type I is a transverse fracture through the physis.
- Type II is a fracture through the physis with a metaphyseal fragment.
- Type III is a fracture through the physis and into the epiphysis (intra-articular).

- Type IV is a fracture through the epiphysis, physis and metaphysis.
- Type V is a crush injury through the physis.

Type I and II have an excellent prognosis, although complete or partial growth arrest may occur in displaced fractures. Type II and III have a worse prognosis, as growth arrest and angular deformity are common problems. Type V fractures have a poor prognosis.

Repeated reduction attempts may increase the incidence of growth plate injuries. Complications unique to paediatric fractures include growth arrest, angular or rotational deformities and osteonecrosis.

Mechanism of injury

Because of structural differences, paediatric fractures tend to occur at lower energies than do adult fractures. Most are a result of compression, torsion, or bending movements. Compression fractures are found at the metaphyseal/ diaphyseal junction and are referred to as 'buckle' or 'torus' fractures. 'Greenstick fractures' occur when the bone is plastically deformed.

Clinical evaluation and investigations

Paediatric trauma patients should undergo a full trauma evaluation. The ABCs are the same as those for adults. Keen diagnostic skills are required when treating children as they are typically not good historians and the parents may not have been present at the time of injury and cannot provide an accurate history. Young children cannot always localise the injury so it is important to evaluate the entire extremity.

Anteroposterior and lateral views of the involved bone and the joint proximal and distal to the suspected area of injury should always be taken. 'Soft signs', such as the fat pad sign should also be looked for closely. CT scan is an option, but one must remember that in paediatric cases compliance will be low and a general anaesthetic may be required to obtain good quality images.

General principles of fracture treatment in children

Fracture reduction should be performed under sedation or a general anaesthetic. Immobilisation should be in a cast that is split to accommodate extremity swelling. All fractures should be elevated at heart level, iced and frequently monitored for any distal neurovascular deficit or development of compartment syndrome.

Few fractures in children require open reduction and internal fixation. If it is necessary, then certain principles should be followed. Repositioning of fragments should be in an anatomical position, otherwise the resulting offset

Table 2.1. Injuries suggestive of child abuse

High specificity	Posterior rib fractures
	Sternal fractures
	Scapular fractures
	Spinous process avulsion fractures
Moderate specificity	Multiple fractures
	Fractures in various stages of healing
	Vertebral compression fractures
	Epiphyseal separations

will cause a bony bridge and joint incongruity. Fixation should be used that can be removed readily. Smooth pins should be used rather than threaded pins and fixation should not cross the physis wherever possible. The placement of compression screws across epiphyseal fragments, parallel to the physis, is an effective means of restoring stable articular congruity. Unnecessary drill holes should be avoided as they may later become iatrogenic fractures. Absorbable sutures should be used to avoid distress to the child on removal of sutures.

Child abuse (non-accidental injury)

More than a million children each year are victims of abuse or neglect and the incidence is increasing (or cases are being better recognised). Approximately one third of abused children are eventually seen by orthopaedic surgeons. A high index of suspicion is needed to make the diagnosis. The highest percentage of child abuse occurs between birth and 2 years of age with neglect being more common than abuse. Children of all socioeconomic backgrounds suffer physical abuse or neglect; however, the incidence does seem to be related to family income. Children with the highest risk of abuse include first-born, unplanned, premature and stepchildren. Children with an increased risk of abuse include children in a single-parent home, children of parents who abuse drugs, children of parents who were abused, children of unemployed parents, and children of families of lower economic status.

Non-accidental injury is most common in children under the age of 3 years. Approximately one third of abused children are eventually seen by an orthopaedic surgeon. An unusual or questionable history or the finding of multiple skin bruises or burns should alert the doctor to the possibility of child abuse. Knowledge of the injury patterns suggestive of non-accidental injury in children is essential (*Table 2.1*). The most common locations (but least specific) for fractures in child abuse are the humerus, tibia and femur.

The differential diagnosis in cases of suspected child abuse include true accidental injury, osteogenesis imperfecta and metabolic disease.

Skeletal survey is a useful initial imaging modality. Nuclear medicine bone scanning may be helpful when the skeletal survey is negative.

Key points

- Children's bones are more malleable and more biologically active with a thick vascular periosteum.
- Children's bones remodel to a greater extent than do adults', so a greater amount of angulation and displacement is acceptable in children.
- Rotational deformities do not remodel acceptably and should be avoided.
- The closer the fracture is to the joint (physes), the better the deformity is tolerated.
- As a general rule, the younger the patient, the greater the potential for remodelling.
- The physes are weak links in the growing skeleton and account for the difference between the location of fractures in children and adults.
- Complications of physeal injuries include limb length discrepancies, angular deformities, malunions and physeal arrest.
- A high index of suspicion is needed to diagnose non-accidental injury.

Further reading

Beaty JH (1997) Orthopaedic aspects of child abuse. *Curr Opin Pediatr* **9**: 100–3

Currey J, Butler G (1975) The mechanical properties of bone tissue in children. *J Bone Joint Surg* **57A**: 810–14

Landin LA (1983) Fracture patterns in children. *Acta Orthop Scand* **54(Suppl 202)**: 1–109

CHAPTER 3

Diagnosis and immediate care of open fractures

Daren Forward, Sam Oussedik and Christopher Moran

Introduction

Any fracture in which the fracture haematoma communicates with the outside world is an 'open fracture'. All open fractures must be treated as a surgical emergency with a clear treatment protocol using a team approach. The accident and emergency (A & E) department forms the initial part of that team. The guiding principles for the team are to prevent infection, unite the fracture and restore function – it is in the first of these that A & E plays an important role. The A & E team will also need an understanding of subsequent management to ensure good initial treatment and communication with the orthopaedic surgeons, patient and relatives.

Surgical debridement of the wound should be performed in the operating theatre, ideally within six hours of injury. Just as important as the timing of surgery is that appropriate surgeons are present, which usually means the involvement of plastic surgeons. Time saved by good management in the A & E department is therefore critical. The timeframe is set by the rapid increase in bacterial counts within the wound. Two-thirds of open fractures are contaminated with bacteria (*Table 3.1*). A bacterial count of more than 100000/g is required to cause infection. The bacterial count rises from 100/g at 2 hours to more than 100000/g at around 5 hours.

Classification

An understanding of the classification of open fractures gives an indication of the severity of injury and the risk of infection and loss of limb (*Table 3.2*). In A & E it provides a guide to the choice of antibiotic prophylaxis. Type I injuries should not be treated with any less urgency than type III injuries.

Initial management

Open fractures are associated with major trauma in 30% of cases (Gustilo *et al*, 1990). Any patient with an open fracture should be managed according to

Table 3.1. Bacterial contamination in open fractures

	n	positive cultures (%)
Gustilo and Anderson (1976)	158	110 (70)
Patzakis and Ivler (1977)	581	356 (62)
Kreder and Armstrong (1994)	86	53 (63)

Table 3.2. Classification of open fractures

Type I	Simple fracture, wound <1cm
Type II	Simple fracture, wound >1cm
Type III	Complex fracture, even with apparently small puncture wound. Soft tissue reconstruction required
Type IIIA	Adequate soft tissue cover
Type IIIB	Soft tissue loss with exposed bone
Type IIIC	Arterial injury requiring repair

From Gustilo and Anderson (1976); Gustilo *et al* (1984)

Advanced Trauma Life Support (ATLS) principles in the first instance. A full primary survey with simultaneous resuscitation and treatment of any possible life-threatening injuries forms the first step in the management of an open fracture. *Table 3.3* gives the mechanisms of injury.

Only when the patient is stable should the fracture be addressed. A thorough secondary survey will detect less obvious injuries in addition to the open fracture. X-rays can be taken at this stage.

Primary soft tissue management

The aim is to achieve an environment around the fracture that is free of bacteria and that prevents further contamination. For all open fractures the following steps should be followed:

- Control haemorrhage using direct pressure.
- Remove gross contamination.
- Photograph wound.
- Apply a sterile dressing.
- Check the neurovascular status of the injured limb.
- Realign and splint the fracture (with adequate analgesia).

Table 3.3. Aetiology of open fractures

Cause	Frequency
Motorcycle	28%
Car	24%
Fall	13%
Pedestrian/car	12%
Crush	8%
Other	15%

From Dellinger *et al* (1988)

- Recheck the neurovascular status.
- Administer intravenous antibiotics and tetanus prophylaxis.

The wound should not be disturbed again until the patient is taken to the operating theatre for further management. This reduces contamination.

Antibiotics

One of the three principal aims is to prevent infection. The basic steps outlined above cannot be missed but antibiotics must be given. Approximately two-thirds of open fractures are contaminated at the time of injury. The choice of antibiotic will be dictated by local policy and advice from the microbiologists, but the following principles may be helpful.

- Always give a cephalosporin (cephradine 1g is used in the authors' centre).
- Add gentamicin for type IIIB and IIIC injuries.
- Add penicillin for farmyard injuries to cover *Clostridium perfringens*.

Tetanus prophylaxis

The disease is caused by tetanospasmin, an exotoxin of the anaerobic gram-positive rod, *Clostridium tetani*. This organism is widespread and grows well in wounds containing necrotic tissue. Prophylaxis should follow the Department of Health guidelines (1996) summarised in *Table 3.4*.

If the patient was not previously immunised and a course is commenced arrangements should be made for the general practitioner to complete this.

Table 3.4. Need for tetanus prophylaxis

	Simple wound	Tetanus-prone wound
Full course + booster within 10 years	Nil required	TTB
Full course + booster more than 10 years ago	TTB	TTB + HATI
Not immunised/unknown	TTB	TTB + HATI

From Department of Health (1996). HATI = 250 units intramuscular human anti-tetanus immunoglobulin administered at a separate site to the booster; TTB = 0.5ml tetanus toxoid booster

Neurovascular complications

Neurovascular complications must be actively excluded and the presence of pulses, motor and sensory function clearly recorded in the notes. If distal perfusion is in doubt the opinion of an orthopaedic and vascular surgeon should be sought urgently. Any arterial injury requiring repair (type IIIC) should be performed with a co-ordinated approach between the orthopaedic and vascular or plastic surgeons.

Nerve injuries generally do not require immediate repair.

Compartment syndrome

Compartment syndrome is tissue hypoxia caused by an increase in pressure in a closed osseo-fascial space. This must be actively excluded. It is a mistake to assume an open injury has already decompressed the compartment. Pain is the main symptom of compartment syndrome. Ongoing pain after adequate analgesia should alert to this diagnosis. The first clinical sign is pain on passive stretch of muscles within the appropriate compartment. Distal pulses are usually present unless an arterial injury has occurred. Therefore extra vigilance is required in patients with altered conscious levels as a result of head injury, alcohol or drugs. Any constricting bandages or casts should be split down to skin and the limb held level with the heart. Urgent open fasciotomy is required.

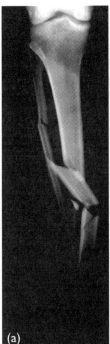
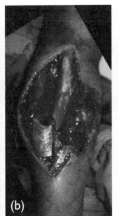
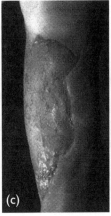
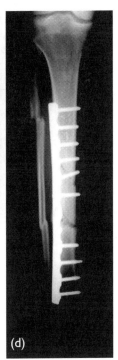

Figure 3.1. (a) Segmental open tibial fracture following motorcycle accident. (b) Wound following primary treatment and debridement – grade IIIB open fracture. (c) After fracture stabilisation the wound was covered by the plastic surgeons with a microvascular free muscle flap and split skin graft. (d) Fracture healing progressing.

Definitive management

The patient will now undergo surgical wound debridement under anaesthesia in the operating theatre. Large volumes of fluid are used to clean the wound and all dead tissue and foreign material must be removed while not jeopardising subsequent soft tissue coverage. In practice, the wound is extended along lines which do not cross neurovascular bundles of local flaps, such that these remain viable for subsequent coverage. The involvement of a plastic surgeon at this first debridement is therefore highly desirable. The fracture will be stabilised with external or internal fixation as this provides the best environment for soft tissue and fracture healing. In general, all open wounds should be left open and the patient returned to theatre at 24–48 hours for repeat surgical debridement and delayed wound closure using direct suture or an appropriate technique from the reconstructive ladder. The patient should remain on antibiotics until definitive wound closure is achieved. *Figure 3.1* illustrates the excellent results that can be achieved.

Conclusions

Osteomyelitis or infected non-union is a disastrous outcome following open fractures. The primary management of the fracture should focus on the prevention of infection. The wound and soft tissues are a very important factor in the management of fractures. Open fractures are a surgical emergency and must be referred early to the orthopaedic trauma team.

Key points

■ Open fractures include all fractures that communicate with the outside world.

■ Open fractures usually result from high energy trauma and may be associated with other significant injuries.

■ They can be classified depending on the size of the soft tissue defect and whether this will close directly.

■ All wounds should be cleansed and photographed prior to being dressed in the emergency department.

■ Rapid involvement of the appropriate surgical team will help to reduce chances of infection and optimise outcome.

■ Joint care from both plastic and orthopaedic surgeons is often required.

References

Dellinger EP, Miller SD, Wertz MJ, Grypma M, Droppert B, Anderson PA (1988) Risk of infection after open fracture of the arm or leg. *Arch Surg* **123**: 1320–7.

Department of Health (1996) *Immunisation against Infectious Diseases*. HMSO, London.

Gustilo RB, Anderson JT (1976) Prevention of infection in the treatment of 1025 open fractures of long bones: Retrospective and prospective analyses. *J Bone Joint Surg Am* **58**: 453–8.

Gustilo RB, Mendoza RM, Williams DN (1984) Problems in the management of type III (severe) open fractures: A new classification of type III open fractures. *J Trauma* **24**: 742–6.

Gustilo RB, Merkow RL, Templeman D (1990) The management of open fractures. *J Bone Joint Surg Am* **72**: 299–304.

Kreder HJ, Armstrong P (1994) The significance of perioperative cultures in open pediatric lower-extremity fractures. *Clin Orthop* **302**: 206–12.

Patzakis MJ, Ivler D (1977) Antibiotic and bacteriologic considerations in open fractures. *South Med J* **70(Suppl 1)**: 46–8.

CHAPTER 4

Compartment syndromes

Rahul Patel and Fares Haddad

Introduction

Compartment syndrome occurs when pressure within a closed muscle compartment exceeds the perfusion pressure and results in muscle and nerve ischaemia. Two distinct conditions are recognised: acute and chronic (exertional) compartment syndromes. Differences in aetiology, pathophysiology and management are elaborated on in this chapter.

Acute compartment syndrome

Acute compartment syndrome (ACS) is a condition that occurs when increased tissue pressure within a myofascial compartment (*Figure 4.1*) compromises the vascular supply and the function of structures within that space. A prerequisite for the development of increased tissue pressure is an envelope restricting the volume available to the enclosed tissue. Such envelopes include the epimysium, the fascia, the skin, and casts or other circumferential dressings.

The increase of hydrostatic and osmotic pressure in the anatomical compartment leads to increased local venous pressure that results in a decrease in the arteriovenous gradient and a subsequent decrease in arterial inflow. A cascade of injury follows, with disruption of the metabolic processes of the muscle, cytolysis, and the release of osmotically active cell contents. This results in further extravasation of fluid from capillaries and added pressure (on the structures) within the compartment, compromising the function of structures such as blood vessels and nerves and the end muscle units they supply.

Aetiology

von Volksmann (1872) suggested that paralysis and contracture of limbs 'too tightly bandaged' resulted from ischaemic change of the muscles. Matsen (1975) suggested that this might be the result of either decreased compartment size or increased compartmental contents. Decreased compartment size may be the result of localised external pressure (eg. a tight dressing), or closure of fascial defects. Increased compartmental contents may result from bleeding (eg. vascular injury, bleeding disorders), capillary permeability (post-ischaemic

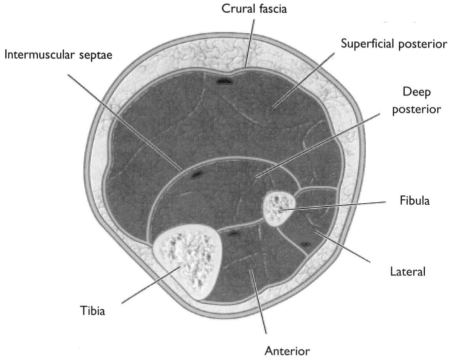

Figure 4.1. Compartments of the lower limb.

swelling, exercise, trauma, burns, intra-arterial drugs) or capillary pressure (exercise, venous obstruction, muscle hypertrophy, infiltration of infusions, nephrotic syndrome).

Fractures are the cause in some 75% of cases, and of these, fractures of the tibia are most commonly responsible. Comminuted fractures are more likely to give rise to ACS and this probably reflects the greater degree of force required to cause this type of injury. Indeed any high energy trauma is more liable to cause ACS, and penetrating injuries such as gunshot wounds often cause severe muscle laceration and arterial tears, which in turn lead to increased intracompartmental pressure. ACS has been recorded in patients with no history of trauma, although such cases appear to be extremely uncommon (Vanneste *et al*, 2003).

It must be borne in mind that ACS can affect the hand, foot, forearm, thigh, lower leg and, rarely, the abdomen.

Pathophysiology

Ischaemia

There are three theories about the development of ischaemia:

* It is the result of arterial spasm caused by increased compartment pressure.
* The theory of critical closing pressure. Because of the small diameter and high mural tension in the arterioles, a significant transmural pressure difference (arteriolar pressure – tissue pressure) is required to maintain patency. If tissue pressure increases or arteriolar pressure decreases so that this difference does not exist, ie. critical closing pressure is reached, they will close (Burton, 1951)
* Because of their thin walls, veins will collapse if tissue pressure exceeds venous pressure. If blood continues to flow from capillaries, the venous pressure continues to increase until it exceeds the tissue pressure and venous drainage is re-established. However, this reduces the arteriovenous gradient and reduces arterial inflow.

Response of muscle to ischaemia

Histamine-like substances are released that dilate the capillary bed and increase endothelial permeability. This leads to intramuscular transudation of plasma with red cell sludging and decreased microcirculation. The muscle gains weight (up to 50% increase). Muscles tolerate 4 hours of ischaemia well, but by 6 hours results are uncertain and after 8 hours, the damage is irreversible (Whitesides and Heckman, 1996).

Diagnosis

In the conscious patient, the main clinical features of ACS are divided into early and late signs and symptoms.

Early

These include pain, disproportionate to the trauma to that limb, aggravated by passive muscle stretching, palpable tightness and tenderness of the compartment, and sensory deficit in the distribution of any sensory nerve traversing the involved compartment.

Late

Paraesthesia, weakness of the muscles and pulselessness are late signs and should not be waited for.

ACS is a clinical diagnosis that can be confirmed by measuring the compartment pressure. There are single use probes available but one can be fashioned using a 14G cannula with slit holes in the tip and an arterial line manometer, the commonest manometer available in anaesthetic rooms. A difference of less than 30mmHg between tissue pressure and the diastolic pressure indicates the need for fasciotomy (McQueen, 1998).

Treatment

Once diagnosis has been made, sensible recommendations have been made by Mars and Hadley (1998). The patient should be kept normotensive as hypotension reduces perfusion pressure and facilitates further tissue injury. Circumferential bandages should be removed. The limb should be maintained at the level of the heart, as elevation reduces the arteriovenous pressure gradient on which perfusion depends, and oxygen should be administered. If a plaster of Paris cast has been applied, this should be split immediately as compartmental pressure falls by 30% when a cast is split on one side and by 65% when the cast is spread after splitting. Splitting the padding reduces it by a further 10% and complete removal of cast by another 15% (Garfin *et al*, 1981).

Fasciotomy is the definitive and only treatment for ACS. Morbidity from delay is significant and so fasciotomy should be performed immediately (Finkelstein *et al*, 1996). Thorough debridement of all non-viable tissue including skin should be carried out.

Fasciotomy is associated with a minor risk of wound infection but limb loss and death results from persisting ischaemia, muscle necrosis and multiorgan failure, not from infection of fasciotomy wounds (Rush *et al*, 1989).

Knowledge of the compartments of the affected limb is paramount to ensure an effective surgical procedure, and fasciotomies should routinely be left open and assessed again in theatre 48 hours later. Primary closure is often difficult and split-skin grafting is frequently necessary. If ACS has existed for more than 8–10 hours, supportive treatment of acute renal failure should be considered.

Complications

The prognosis of ACS depends upon a number of factors. These include most importantly the rapidity with which it is diagnosed and treated, and whether or not complications occur.

Infection is a serious complication of ACS, and is more likely in cases where decompression is delayed. When it occurs, it increases the likelihood of amputation. Systemic complications include renal failure, adult respiratory distress syndrome and disseminated intravascular coagulation.

Untreated ACS results in Volkmann's ischaemic contracture, a disabling deformity of the limb. Cosmetic disfigurement may occur from the surgical procedures involved in treatment.

Chronic compartment syndrome

Chronic compartment syndrome (CCS), also known as exertional compartment syndrome, is characterised by exertional limb pain, swelling and dysaesthesia during and immediately after exercise. It is mostly seen in athletes and military recruits. The pain gradually worsens as exercise continues, ultimately restricting performance.

Although this condition usually involves the lower limb, rare cases do occur in which the upper limb is primarily affected, eg. in weightlifters. Upper limb symptoms may be reproducible at a specific workload or time interval. Symptoms generally subside within an hour or so of stopping the activity but recur when exercise is resumed.

Muscle weakness of the affected limb may be a feature of these episodes and gradually increasing fullness is a frequent complaint. Pain is increased both on passive stretching and active contraction.

The clinical features of CCS are only evident in the immediate aftermath of exercise, and the nature and location of signs and symptoms will depend on the compartment affected.

Pathophysiology

The pathogenesis of this condition is uncertain, although it probably resembles that of ACS in that structures within a closed myofascial compartment are compressed. During exercise, muscle bulk increases some 20% and, allied with repetitive muscle contraction, may increase intracompartmental pressure to a level that causes transient ischaemia and deoxygenation (Mohler *et al*, 1997).

Symptoms of CCS probably occur when the pressure between successive muscle contractions remains high within a small unyielding fascial compartment (Schissel and Godwin, 1999).

An alternative explanation is that muscle tissue, damaged by repetitive hard surface exercise, releases protein-bound ions which increase osmotic pressure, provoke oedema and so decrease blood flow within the compartment.

The predisposing factors and pathophysiology of CCS are imperfectly understood and although cases have been reported in which the condition appears to have originated at the time of some minor trauma, such instances appear to be rare (Tubb and Vermillion, 2001).

Each compartment of the leg contains one major nerve. The anterior compartment contains the deep peroneal nerve, the lateral compartment contains the superficial peroneal nerve, the deep posterior compartment contains the posterior tibial nerve and the superficial posterior compartment contains the sural nerve. When the pressure in a compartment increases, the vascular supply to the nerves can be affected causing paraesthesia to occur.

Diagnosis

No abnormalities are usually evident unless the patient is seen immediately after exercise.

Muscle atrophy may be noticed. Tenderness and increased tension in the involved compartment is frequently present. Tenderness directly over the tibia, however, is more characteristic of a stress fracture, tibialis posterior tendonitis or periostitis.

Passive stretching of the involved muscle after exercise may increase pain. The key to diagnosis is compartment pressure measurements. A resting pressure must be measured first which is then followed by exercise, during which sequential measurements are taken at specific time intervals, culminating in final readings 5, 10 and 20 minutes after exercise to ensure pressure has returned to baseline. It is very important that symptoms are elicited during this process and measurements taken at intervals until they subside. A positive indication of CCS is post-exercise pressures in excess of their insertional pressure and/or pressures in excess of 15mmHg persisting for longer than 15 minutes. Definitions for elevated pressures are pre-exercise: >14–15mmHg; 1 minute post-exercise: >30mmHg; 5 minutes post-exercise: >19–20mmHg.

Treatment

Although there have been reports of successful treatment of CCS by conservative means, massage and physiotherapy alone are rarely satisfactory and fasciotomy is the treatment of choice (Brennan and Kane, 2003; Fraipont and Adamson, 2003).

Surgical intervention has a generally satisfactory outcome (Turnipseed, 2002) with some 70–85% of patients able to return to pre-treatment levels of activity without symptoms. The success rate depends largely on the compartment concerned, and patients with lower limb CCS in whom the deep posterior compartment is affected respond less well than those whose anterior or lateral compartment is involved. Cases of recurrent CCS have been reported, almost certainly attributable to scarring and closure of the initial compartment release.

Complications

Complications including inability to return to pre-morbid performance levels, weakness in muscles of the affected compartment and recurrence of symptoms may be noticed.

Conclusions

ACS and CCS may have linked pathophysiology but they occur in very different clinical settings. ACS is usually associated with a fracture but not exclusively. It is a serious limb-threatening condition and delay in treatment of ACS increases morbidity and complications. ACS can occur in open fracture injuries.

CCS most commonly affects the lower extremities in competitive athletes, and is probably caused by raised pressure within a non-compliant myofascial compartment as a result of repetitive muscle activity, causing symptoms during and immediately after exercise. Diagnosis is more complicated but less urgent than ACS.

Key points

- Acute compartment syndrome is a condition that occurs when increased tissue pressure within a myofascial compartment compromises the vascular supply and the function of structures within that space.
- Acute compartment syndrome can affect the hand, foot, forearm, thigh, lower leg and rarely the abdomen; fractures are the cause in some 75% of cases.
- Diagnosis of acute compartment syndrome is mainly a clinical one which may be supported by compartment pressure measurement.
- Chronic compartment syndrome is characterised by exertional limb pain, swelling and dysaesthesia during and immediately after exercise.
- Diagnosis of chronic compartment syndrome is both clinical, mainly from the history, and physical examination, and from compartment pressure measurements before, during and after exercise.

References

Brennan FH, Kane SF (2003) Diagnosis, treatment options, and rehabilitation of chronic lower leg exertional compartment syndrome. *Curr Sports Med Rep* **2**(5): 247–50.

Burton AC (1951) On the physical equilibrium of small blood vessels. *Am J Physiol* **164**: 319–29.

Finkelstein JA, Hunter GA, Hu RW (1996) Lower limb compartment syndrome: course after delayed fasciotomy. *J Trauma* **40**(3): 342–4.

Fraipont MJ, Adamson GJ (2003) Chronic exertional compartment syndrome. *J Am Acad Orthop Surg* **11**(4): 268–76.

Garfin SR, Mubarak SJ, Evans KL, Hargen AR, Akeson WH (1981) Quantification of intracompartmental pressure and volume under plaster casts. *JBJS* **63A**: 449–53.

Mars M, Hadley GP (1998) Raised intracompartmental pressure and compartment syndromes. *Injury* **29**(6): 403–11.

Matsen FA 3rd (1975) Compartment syndrome-a unified concept. *Clin Orth* **113**: 8–14.

McQueen M (1998) Acute compartment syndrome. *Acta Chir Belg* **98(4)**: 166–70.

Mohler IR, Styf JR, Pedowitz RA, Hargens AR, Gershuni DH (1997) Intramuscular deoxygenation during exercise in patients who have chronic anterior compartment syndrome of the leg. *JBJS Am* **79(6)**: 844–9.

Rush DS, Frame SB, Bell RM, Berg EE, Kerstein MD, Haynes JL (1989) Does open fasciotomy contribute to morbidity and mortality after acute lower extremity ischemia and revascularization? *J Vasc Surg* **10(3)**: 343–50.

Schissel DJ, Godwin J (1999) Effort-related chronic compartment syndrome of the lower extremity. *Mil Med* **164(11)**: 830–2.

Tubb CC, Vermillion D (2001) Chronic exertional compartment syndrome after minor injury to the lower extremity. *Mil Med* **166(4)**: 366–8.

Turnipseed WD (2002) Diagnosis and management of chronic compartment syndrome. *Surgery* **132(4)**: 613–17.

Vanneste DR, Janzing HM, Broos PL (2003) The acute atraumatic peroneal compartment syndrome, a rare and therefore sometimes unrecognised entity. *Acta Chir Belg* **103(4)**: 355–7.

von Volkmann R (1872) Verletzungen und krannkheiten der bewwgungsorgane. *Handbuch der Allegemeinen und Speziellen Chirurgie* **2**: 234–920.

Whitesides TE, Heckman MM (1996) Acute compartment syndrome: update on diagnosis and treatment. *J Am Acad Orthop Surg* **4(4)**: 209–18.

Section Two:

Regional trauma

CHAPTER 5

The management and treatment of cervical spine injuries

Hesham Al-Khateeb and Sam Oussedik

Introduction

The cervical spine is a complex and fragile musculoskeletal structure. Important neurological, vascular, respiratory and gastrointestinal structures traverse the cervical region. Injuries to the cervical spine can produce a wide spectrum of clinical presentations. Early recognition of potential cervical spine trauma is vital for optimal functional outcome. Appropriate protective and diagnostic interventions need to be instituted in an efficient and timely manner to maximise treatment results and minimise adverse outcomes. Recent advances in resuscitation techniques, imaging modalities, and surgical technique, together with the establishment of regional trauma care systems, have enabled clinicians to maximise patients' chances of functional recovery from spinal cord injuries and to minimise risks of secondary injury.

Anatomy

Most cervical spine fractures occur predominantly at one of two levels, one third of injuries occurring at the level of C2, and one half of injuries occurring at the level of C6 or C7. Most fatal cervical spine injuries occur in upper cervical levels, either at the craniocervical junction, C1 or C2.

The normal anatomy of the cervical spine consists of seven cervical vertebrae separated by intervertebral discs and joined by a complex network of ligaments. This structure allows the individual bony elements to behave as a single unit.

The cervical spine can be divided into three distinct columns (*Figure 5.1*): anterior, middle, and posterior. The anterior column is composed of two thirds of the vertebral bodies, the annulus fibrosis, intervertebral discs, and the anterior longitudinal ligament. The middle column is composed of the posterior third of the vertebral bodies, the annulus, the intervertebral disc, and posterior longitudinal ligament. The posterior column contains all of the remaining

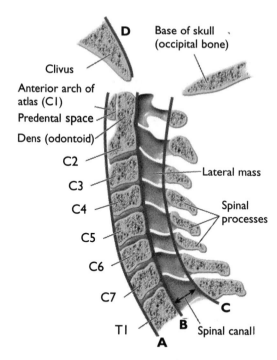

Figure 5.1. The divisions of the cervical spine. A: anterior; B: middle; C: posterior columns.

posterior elements formed by the pedicles, transverse processes, articulating facets, laminae, and spinous processes.

The atlas C1 and the axis C2 differ markedly from other cervical vertebrae. The atlas has no vertebral body; it is composed of a thick anterior arch with two prominent lateral masses and a thin posterior arch. The axis includes the odontoid process that represents fused remnants of the atlas body. The odontoid process is held in tight approximation to the posterior aspect of the anterior arch of C1 by the transverse ligament, which stabilises the atlanto-axial joint.

Classification

Cervical spine injuries are best classified by considering the mechanism of injury. This includes:

- flexion
- flexion-rotation
- extension
- extension-rotation
- vertical compression
- lateral flexion
- imprecisely understood mechanisms that may result in odontoid fractures and atlanto-occipital dislocation.

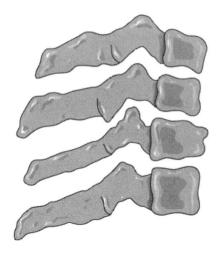

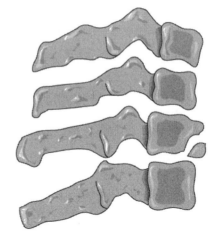

Figure 5.2. Simple wedge fracture.

Figure 5.3. Flexion teardrop fracture.

Flexion injuries

Simple wedge fracture

With a pure flexion injury, a longitudinal pull is exerted on the strong nuchal ligament complex which usually remains intact (*Figure 5.2*). The prevertebral soft tissues appear swollen. The posterior column remains intact, making this a stable fracture that requires only the use of a cervical orthosis for treatment.

Flexion teardrop fracture

A flexion teardrop fracture occurs when flexion of the spine, along with vertical axial compression, causes a fracture of the antero-inferior aspect of the vertebral body (*Figure 5.3*). This injury involves disruption of all three columns, making it an extremely unstable fracture that frequently is associated with spinal cord injury. Initial management is application of traction with cervical tongs.

Anterior subluxation

Anterior subluxation in the cervical spine occurs when posterior ligamentous complexes (nuchal ligament, capsular ligaments, ligamenta flava, posterior longitudinal ligament) rupture (*Figure 5.4*). As the anterior columns remain intact, this fracture is considered mechanically stable by definition.

Bilateral facet dislocation

Bilateral facet dislocation is an extreme form of anterior subluxation that occurs when a significant degree of flexion and anterior subluxation causes ligamentous disruption to extend anteriorly, causing significant anterior

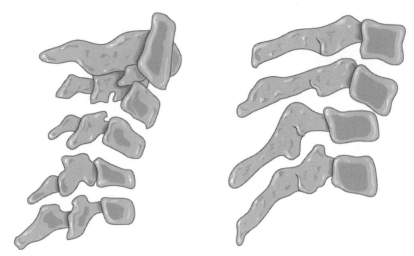

Figure 5.4. Anterior facet dislocation.   Figure 5.5. Bilateral facet dislocation.

displacement of the spine at the level of injury (*Figure 5.5*). This is an extremely unstable condition and is associated with a high prevalence of spinal cord injuries. Initial management is closed reduction and traction with cervical tongs.

'Clay shoveller' fracture

Abrupt flexion of the neck, combined with a heavy upper body and lower neck muscular contraction, results in an oblique fracture of the base of the spinous process, which is avulsed by the intact and powerful supraspinous ligament (*Figure 5.6*).

Injury is commonly observed in a lateral view, since the avulsed fragment is readily evident. Injury commonly occurs in lower cervical vertebrae; visualisation of the C7–T1 junction in the lateral view is therefore imperative.

Since injury involves only the spinous process, this fracture is considered stable, and it is not associated with neurological impairment. Management involves only cervical immobilisation for comfort.

Flexion-rotation injuries

Unilateral facet dislocation

Unilateral facet dislocation occurs when flexion and rotation combine to force one inferior articular facet of an upper vertebra to pass superior and anterior to the superior articular facet of a lower vertebra, coming to rest in the intervertebral foramen (*Figure 5.7*). Although the posterior ligament is disrupted, vertebrae are locked in place, making this injury stable. The injury is seldom associated with neurological deficit.

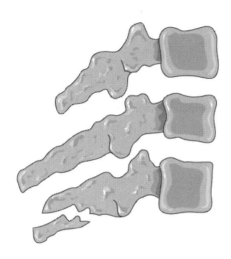

Figure 5.6. The 'Clay-Shoveller' fracture.

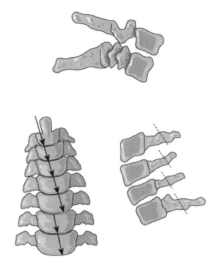

Figure 5.7. Unilateral facet dislocation.

Rotary atlanto-axial dislocation

This injury is a specific type of unilateral facet dislocation. Radiographically, the odontoid view shows asymmetry of the lateral masses of C1 with respect to the dens along with unilateral magnification of a lateral mass of C1 (wink sign). This injury is considered unstable because of its location.

Extension injuries

Hangman fracture

The hangman fracture is a traumatic spondylolisthesis of C2 (*Figure 5.8*). In the past this type of fracture resulted from hanging, although nowadays road traffic accidents are a

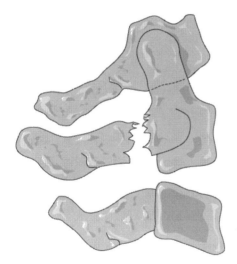

Figure 5.8. The Hangman fracture.

more common cause. Bilateral fractures through the pedicles of C2 result from hyperextension.

Although considered an unstable fracture, it is seldom associated with spinal injury, since the anteroposterior diameter of the spinal canal is greatest at this level, and the fractured pedicles allow decompression. When associated with unilateral or bilateral facet dislocation at the level of C2, this particular type of hangman fracture is unstable and has a high rate of neurological complications that require immediate cervical traction

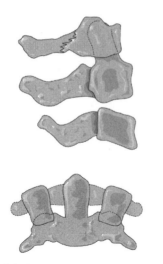

Figure 5.9. Posterior neural arch fracture.

to reduce the facet dislocation. All other types of hangman fracture can be managed initially with cervical immobilisation.

Extension teardrop fracture

As with flexion teardrop fracture, extension teardrop fracture also manifests with a displaced antero-inferior bony fragment. This fracture occurs when the anterior longitudinal ligament pulls a fragment away from the inferior aspect of the vertebra because of sudden hyperextension.

The fracture is common after diving accidents and tends to occur at lower cervical levels. It may also be associated with the central cord syndrome as a result of buckling of the ligamenta flava into the spinal canal during the hyperextension phase of the injury.

This injury is stable in flexion but highly unstable in extension. Initial management is avoidance of iatrogenic extension and cervical traction with tongs.

Posterior neural arch fracture

This is a fracture of the posterior arch of C1 (posterior neural arch fracture) (*Figure 5.9*). This fracture occurs when the head is hyperextended and the posterior neural arch of C1 is compressed between the occiput and the strong and prominent spinous process of C2, causing the weak posterior arch of C1 to fracture.

The transverse ligament and the anterior arch of C1 are not involved, making this fracture stable. Initial management involves the differentiation of this benign fracture from a Jefferson fracture. Once this is accomplished, the use of a cervical collar suffices.

Vertical (axial) compression injuries

Jefferson fracture

This is a burst fracture of the ring of C1 (*Figure 5.10*).

This fracture is caused by a compressive downward force that is transmitted evenly through the occipital condyles to the superior articular surfaces of the lateral masses of C1. This process displaces the masses laterally and causes fractures of the anterior and posterior arches, along with possible disruption

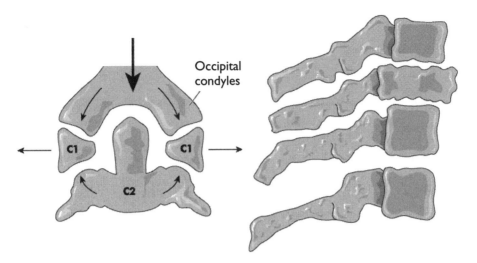

Figure 5.10. Pathophysiology of the Jefferson fracture.

Figure 5.11. Burst fracture of the vertebral body.

of the transverse ligament. Quadruple fracture of all four aspects of the C1 ring occurs.

When displacement of the lateral masses is more than 6.9mm, complete disruption of the transverse ligament has occurred, and immediate cervical traction is warranted. If displacement is less than 6.9mm, the transverse ligament is still competent and neurological injury is unlikely.

Burst fracture of the vertebral body

When downward compressive force is transmitted to lower levels in the cervical spine, the body of the cervical vertebra can shatter outward, causing a burst fracture (*Figure 5.11*). This fracture involves disruption of the anterior and middle columns, with a variable degree of posterior protrusion of the latter.

Burst fractures require assessment by axial computed tomography (CT) scan or magnetic resonance imaging (MRI) to document the amount of middle column retropulsion.

Burst fractures with a loss in height of more than 25%, retropulsion, or neurological deficit can be managed initially by the application of traction with cervical tongs. In the absence of these features, the fracture is considered stable.

Mechanism of injury, location and clinical relevance

Upper cervical spine (occiput to C2) injuries

Injuries at the upper cervical level are considered unstable because of their location. Nevertheless, since the diameter of the spinal canal is greatest at the level of C2, spinal cord injury from compression is the exception rather than the rule. Incompletely understood mechanisms or a combination of them usually produce injuries encountered at this level. Common injuries include the following.

Atlas (C1) fractures

Four types of atlas fractures result from impaction of the occipital condyles on the atlas, causing single or multiple fractures around the ring.

The first two types of atlas fracture are stable and include isolated fractures of the anterior and posterior arch of C1 respectively (posterior arch fracture is described under extension injury).

Initial management of types I, II, and III atlas fractures consists of the application of a cervical collar. The type IV or Jefferson fracture is managed with cervical traction.

Atlanto-axial subluxation

When flexion occurs without a lateral or rotatory component at the upper cervical level, it can cause an anterior dislocation at the atlanto-axial joint if the transverse ligament is disrupted. Since the transverse ligament is the main stabilising force of the atlanto-axial joint, this injury is unstable.

Neurological injury may occur from cord compression between the odontoid process and posterior arch of C1.

Atlanto-occipital dislocation

When severe flexion or extension exists at the upper cervical level, atlanto-occipital dislocation may occur. Atlanto-occipital dislocation involves complete disruption of all ligamentous relationships between the occiput and the atlas. Death usually occurs immediately from stretching of the brainstem, which causes respiratory arrest.

Cervical traction is absolutely contraindicated, since further stretching of the brainstem can occur.

Odontoid process fractures

The three types of odontoid process fractures are classified. The classification is based on the anatomical level at which the fracture occurs (*Table 5.1* and *Figure 5.12*).

With types II and III fractures, the fractured segment may be displaced anteriorly, laterally, or posteriorly. Since posterior displacement of segment is more common, the prevalence of spinal cord injury is as high as 10% with these fractures.

Initial management of a type I dens fracture is use of a cervical collar. Management of types II and III is by applying traction with cervical tongs.

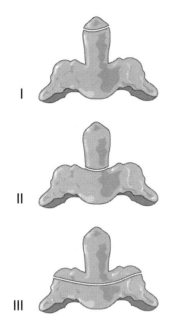

I

II

III

Figure 5.12. Odontoid process fracture.

Table 5.1. Classification of odontoid process fractures

Type I	Odontoid fracture is an avulsion of the tip of the dens at the insertion site of the alar ligament
Type II	Fractures occur at the base of the dens and are the most common odontoid fractures
Type III	Odontoid fracture occurs when the fracture line extends into the body of the axis

Occipital condyle fracture

Occipital condyle fractures are caused by a combination of vertical compression and lateral bending. These fractures are associated with significant head trauma and usually are accompanied by cranial nerve deficits.

These mechanically stable injuries require only immobilisation for management, and most heal uneventfully. These fractures are significant because of other associated injuries.

Whiplash injuries

The whiplash syndrome is a collection of symptoms produced by a soft tissue injury of the cervical spine. It often occurs following a rear-end automobile collision.

Mechanism of injury

The most common cause of whiplash injury is a rear-end impact in an automobile accident. The crash causes the trunk to accelerate in a forward direction and the unsupported head cannot follow this motion, resulting in hyperextension beyond the normal range of 60°.

Table 5.2. The Gargan and Bannister classification

Grade A	No symptoms
Grade B	Nuisance symptoms but which do not interfere with occupation or leisure
Grade C	Intrusive symptoms requiring intermittent analgesia, orthotics or physical therapy
Grade D	Disabling symptoms requiring time off work and regular analgesia, orthotics, and repeated medical consultation

Classification

Several classification systems exist, most commonly based on symptom severity. Both the Neck Disability Index and the Gargan and Bannister classification (*Table 5.2*) (Khan *et al*, 2002) utilise the impact patients' symptoms have on their lifestyle.

Clinical picture and investigations

Hyperextension injury can result in a vast array of symptoms. Thirty percent of patients attending hospital after an automobile accident describe neck pain. There is often radiation to the occiput, shoulders, and upper limbs. Low back pain is a symptom often overlooked. Other symptoms include interscapular pain, arm and hand pain, vertigo, auditory problems, and visual problems.

The majority of patients experience discomfort within 2 days of the accident but delayed symptoms occur in 35%. Symptoms are usually disproportionate to the physical signs, the most common being a decreased range of movement in a tender neck but actual nerve deficit is infrequent, seen in 10 of 61 patients in one series (Norris and Watt, 1983).

There is no diagnostic test for whiplash syndrome, and there is a poor correlation between symptoms and findings on plain radiographs, scintigraphy or MRI.

Conventional radiographs have low yield of bone injury – in the absence of high force or high speed impacts, clinicians should feel safe managing patients involved in rear end collisions without the use of radiographs. The use of MRI is indicated only later to investigate patients with persistent neurological deficits or clinical signs of nerve root compression.

Treatment

The treatment of whiplash injury is generally disappointing, and many patients rapidly abandon conventional medicine and seek alternative practitioners. The most common acute treatment consists of a soft collar and physiotherapy, yet evidence (Khan et al, 2002) suggests that these are among the least useful modes of treatment.

In 1996, Lord *et al* identified the zygapophyseal joint as the common basis for chronic neck pain in whiplash injury and treatment is being targeted increasingly at relieving pain from the source.

Conclusion

The region between the occiput and axis is an inherently unstable region but fortunately has a large spinal canal diameter lessening the likelihood of neurological trauma. Strong ligamentous structures provide stability but have poor healing capacity when injured. Immobilisation of the cervical spine by the use of such devices as the halo-vest can be successful in the treatment of many injuries. This uses a series of pins inserted into the cranium which are then secured to a metal ring. This controls head movements. This ring or halo is then attached to a vest which fits securely over the upper part of the thorax. Thus head movements and therefore cervical spine movement can be controlled.

Surgery is warranted in patients with occipito-atlantal instability, transverse ligament disruptions, displaced type II odontoid fractures and rarely in hangman's fractures. Newer surgical techniques increase stability, allowing early mobilisation and avoid the halo-vest.

Whiplash injuries are a common cause of chronic disability. Most cases resolve in weeks or months but about 40% become chronic, and current treatment of patients is inadequate. The future must involve targeting treatments more effectively, either at the specific treatable organic lesion seen in about half of chronic cases, or at the predominantly psychological response to pain seen in the other half.

Key points

- The cervical spine is a relatively vulnerable structure.
- Cervical spine injuries may be complicated by spinal cord injury.
- Routine cervical spine immobilisation of all trauma patients will help minimise further injury.
- Careful assessment and early diagnosis will help to optimise outcome.
- Whiplash injuries are a common cause of chronic disability.
- Combining psychological and physical therapy may be necessary to optimise outcome.

References

Khan S, Gargan M, Bannister G (2002) Whiplash injuries. In: Bulstrode C, Buckwater J, Carr A *et al* (eds) *Oxford Textbook of Orthopaedics and Trauma*. Oxford University Press, Oxford

Lord S, Barnsley L, Wallis B, Bogduk N (1996) Percutaneous radiofrequency neurotomy for chronic cervical zygapophyseal joint pain. *N Engl J Med* **335(23)**: 1721–6

Further reading

Belval E, Roy S (2005) *Fractures, Cervical Spine*. E-Medicine. Available from www.emedicine. com

Davidson JSD, Birdsell DC (1989) Cervical spine injury in patients with facial skeletal trauma. *J Trauma* **29**: 1276–8

Ellis GL (1991) Imaging of the atlas (C1) and axis (C2). *Emerg Med Clin North Am* **9(4)**: 719–32

Hills MW, Deane SA (1993 Head injury and facial injury: Is there an increased risk of cervical spine injury? *J Trauma* **34(4)**: 549–53; discussion 553–4

Hockberger RS, Kirshebaum KJ, Doris PE (1998) Spinal injuries. In: Rosen P, Barkin R, Danzl DF *et al* (eds) *Emergency Medicine: Concepts and Clinical Practice*. 4th edn. Mosby-Year Book, St Louis, USA: 462–503

Ivy ME, Cohn SM (1997) Addressing the myths of cervical spine injury management. *Am J Emerg Med* **15(6)**: 591–5

Jacobs LM, Schwartz R (1986) Prospective analysis of acute cervical spine injury: A methodology to predict injury. *Ann Emerg Med* **15**: 44–9

Jens R, Chapman, Sohail K Mirza, Mark Konadi M (1997) *Emergency Management of the Traumatized Cervical Spine. Oxford textbook of Orthopaedics and Trauma. Advanced Trauma Life Support, Student Course Manual*. Oxford University Press, Oxford

Mahoney BD (1996) Spinal injuries. In: Tintinalli JE, Krone RL, Ruiz E (eds) *Emergency Medicine: A Comprehensive Study Guide*. 4th edn. McGraw Hill Text, New York, USA: 1147–53

National Spinal Cord Injury Statistical Center (NSCISC) (1996) *Spinal Cord Injury. Facts and Figures at a Glance*. NSCISC, Birmingham AL

Norris SH, Watt I (1983) The prognosis of neck injuries resulting from rear-end vehicle collisions. *J Bone Joint Surg Br* **65(5)**: 608–11

O'Malley KF, Ross SE (1988) The incidence of injury to the cervical spine in patients with craniocerebral injury. *J Trauma* **28**: 1476–14

Proudfoot J, Pollack E, Friedland LR (1996) Pediatric cervical spine injury: Navigating the nuances and minimizing complications. *Pediatr Emerg Med Rep* **1(9)**: 83–94

Roberge RJ, Wears RC, Kelly M (1988) Selective application of cervical spine radiography in alert victims of blunt trauma: A prospective study. *J Trauma* **28**: 784–8

Sinclair D, Schwartz M, Gruss J *et al* (1988) A retrospective review of the relationship between facial fractures, head injuries, and cervical spine injuries. *J Emerg Med* **6**: 109–12

Trafton PG (1982) Spinal cord injuries. *Surg Clin North Am* **62(1)**: 61–72

Velmahos GC, Theodorou D, Tatevossian R *et al* (1996) Radiographic cervical spine evaluation in the alert asymptomatic blunt trauma victim: Much ado about nothing. *J Trauma* **40(5)**: 768–74

CHAPTER 6

Injuries to the lumbar spine: Identification and management

Alexander Woolard and Sam Oussedik

Fifteen percent of spinal injuries occur in the lumbosacral region. Damage to the spinal cord or cauda equina is a possible complication. Thorough assessment of all trauma patients for such injuries will result in early diagnosis and optimal outcome can be achieved. This chapter looks at the identification and management of injuries to the lumbar spine.

Injury to the spine must always be actively sought and excluded in any trauma scenario. Approximately 5% of patients with a head injury will have an associated spinal injury and 15% of all spinal injuries occur in the lumbosacral region. A sound understanding of these injuries and their treatments is vital in optimising outcome.

Anatomy

The lumbar spine consists of the five lumbar vertebrae with attached muscles and ligaments, and the spinal cord and cauda equina within a dural sac.

The spinal cord terminates at the inferior border of the L1 vertebral body becoming the cauda equina, which is comprised of sensory and motor nerve roots. These nerve roots have proportionally more room within the bony confines of the spinal canal than the spinal cord in the cervical and thoracic spine, meaning that neurological injury is less likely with lumbar fractures than with injuries at other levels.

It is useful to consider the spine as three columns as described by Denis (1983) (*Figure 6.1*). The three columns are:

- Anterior column – consists of the anterior longitudinal ligament, the anterior half of the vertebral body and annulus.
- Middle column – consists of the posterior longitudinal ligament and the posterior half of the vertebral body and annulus.
- Posterior column – consists of the pedicles, facets, laminae and posterior ligamentous complex (supraspinous, infraspinous, ligamentum flavum and facet joint capsules).

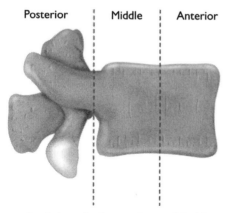

Posterior   Middle   Anterior

Figure 6.1. The spine as three columns (anterior, middle and posterior) as described by Denis (1983).

An injury is deemed unstable if any two of the three columns are involved. However, thoracolumbar injury stability usually follows middle column integrity; if this is intact then the injury is usually stable.

Initial management of trauma

The principles of spinal trauma management are as per Advanced Trauma Life Support (ATLS) protocol. With any suspicion of spinal injury patients should be triple immobilised and strapped to a long spinal board. Any transfers should be conducted by formal log roll until the spine has been cleared by examination and/or X-rays. Standard observations need to be monitored for any sign of neurogenic shock (hypotension without tachycardia or peripheral vasoconstriction) which indicates dysfunction of nervous tissue due to physiological causes.

Triple immobilisation

The cervical spine can only be immobilised manually (*Figure 6.2*) by supporting the head between the arms and fixing in relation to the neck and shoulders or through triple immobilisation using a correctly fitting collar, blocks and tape (*Figure 6.3*). When fixing a patient to a long spinal board or trolley the cervical spine should always be controlled manually until the rest of the body has been secured.

Log roll

The log roll is a method for moving and examining a patient while excluding movement of the spine. It requires a minimum of five people, four to move the patient and one to examine the spine. All directions come from the 'leader' who is responsible for manual control of the cervical spine (*Figure 6.2*). Three people now position themselves along one side of the patient, one responsible

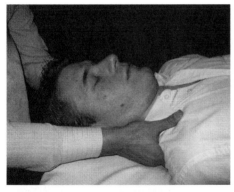

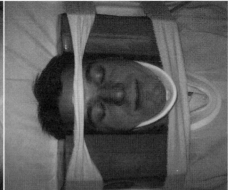

Figure 6.2. To immobilise the cervical spine the head must be supported between the arms and fixed in relation to the neck and shoulders.

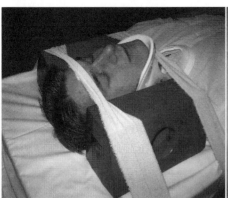

Figure 6.3 Triple immobilisation using collar, blocks and tape.

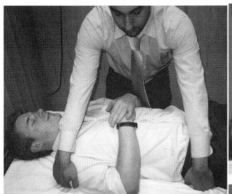

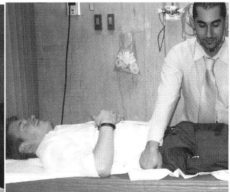

Figure 6.4. Positioning for support of chest and upper limbs.

Figure 6.5. Positioning for support of the pelvis.

for the chest and upper limbs (*Figure 6.4*), one for the pelvis (*Figure 6.5*) and one for the lower limbs (*Figure 6.6*). If there is any suggestion of trauma to one particular side it is sensible to roll onto the unaffected side.

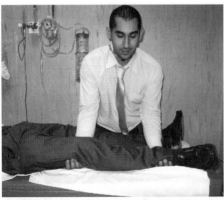

Figure 6.6. Positioning for support of lower limbs.

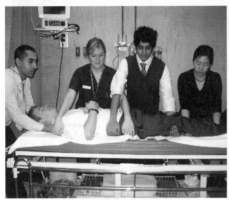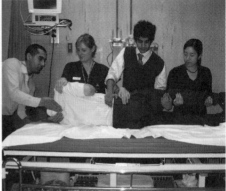

Figure 6.7. (left) 'Ready, brace, roll' position. (right) Patient is rolled 90° towards the team.

The examiner takes up position on the other side of the patient and, provided he or she is conscious, explains the procedure of the examination with particular emphasis on the necessity to answer 'yes' or 'no' as the spine is palpated for bony pain as opposed to nodding agreement.

The leader then announces 'ready, brace, roll' at which point the patient is rolled to 90° towards the team (*Figure 6.7*). The examiner now inspects the spine looking for areas of obvious trauma (eg. contusion, bleeding, laceration) and palpates for any obvious steps or tenderness along every spinous process. The examination is not complete until sacral nerve roots have been assessed by rectal examination for perianal sensation and anal tone.

Mechanisms of injury

Most trauma to the lumbar spine occurs in the context of road traffic accidents and falls from a height. The remainder result from sporting activity or acts of violence.

Table 6.1. Classification of lumbar fractures

Fracture	Anterior	Middle	Posterior
Compression	Compression	None	None/distraction
Burst	Compression	Compression	None/distraction
Flexion/distraction	None/comp.	Distraction	Distraction
Fracture/dislocation	Comp. +/- rotation/shear	Distraction +/- rotation/shear	Distraction +/- rotation/shear

Classification of injuries

The bony architecture of the lumbar spine is normally disrupted in one of four patterns as a result of trauma. These can be summarised according to their effects on the three anatomical columns as described by Denis (1983) (*Table 6.1*).

Compression

This arises as a result of lateral or anterior flexion that produces failure of the anterior column. These injuries are usually stable and rarely cause neurological impairment.

Burst

A burst fracture is commonly associated with a fall from a height and is a result of axial load causing a failure of the vertebral body and disruption of the anterior and middle columns. Burst fractures can be further subdivided into five characteristic patterns (*Figure 6.8*). The five patterns are:

- superior and inferior vertebral body end plates
- superior vertebral body end plate
- inferior vertebral body end plate
- rotational
- lateral wedging of vertebral body.

Flexion/distraction

Classically associated with deceleration forces while restrained by a lap seat-belt fracture/distraction injuries arise from a distracting force across the three columns with the anterior column acting as the centre of rotation. If this only involves

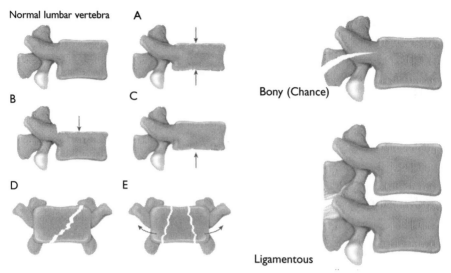

Normal lumbar vertebra   A

B   C

D   E

Bony (Chance)

Ligamentous

Figure 6.8. Five characteristic patterns of
burst fractures. A: Superior and inferior;
B: Superior; C: Inferior vertebral body end
plate; D: Rotational; E: Lateral wedging of
vertebral body.

Figure 6.9. Chance fracture.

osseous structures it is known as a Chance fracture (Chance, 1948), but it may
disrupt any of the ligamentous structures (*Figure 6.9*). Neurological deficit is
only likely to arise if there is a significant degree of translation between affected
segments. If this is the case it is more likely to be a fracture/dislocation injury.

Fracture/dislocation

These injuries show disruption of the bony and ligamentous structures of all
three columns through a combination of compression, rotation, tension and
shear forces. The fracture line can run across the vertebral body or the disc
space. The displacement can occur in posterior-anterior (PA) direction, where
the superior segment slides forwards (as in a heavy load on the back), or an
anterior-posterior (AP) direction. In a PA direction the facets prohibit the
anterior displacement of the posterior arch of the vertebra which subsequently
often fractures in multiple locations and detaches from the lamina. For this
reason dural tears, and neurological injury, are far more common with this
injury than with AP displacement (Bolesta *et al*, 1996).

Neurological injury

Neurological damage from the above can be classified according to the nature
of the insult to the axonal structures.

Contusion

This is responsible for the majority of injuries and constitutes a sudden, but brief increase of pressure on the cord/nerve roots. This is usually irreversible and associated with vascular injury and intramedullary haemorrhage.

Compression

Compression reduces the size of the spinal canal and is normally associated with a translation or angulation deformity (eg. burst injuries and disc herniation). It interferes with both axonal flow and spinal vasculature which can lead to secondary ischaemia and further insult.

Stretch

Stretching occurs with a flexion/distraction injury and leads to capillary and axonal collapse secondary to tensile distortion.

Laceration

Lacerating injuries to the spinal cord can be a result of foreign bodies or bony fragments that occur with a translational fracture through the vertebrae.

Level and extent of injury

In addition to recording the vertebral level of injury it is very important to quantify the degree of neuronal injury since this is a key prognostic indicator. It is vital to ascertain and record whether the injury is complete or incomplete.

A complete injury is one where there is no motor or sensory function caudal to the injury and the bulbocavernosus reflex is intact. If this S3–4 reflex arc is functional spinal shock can be ruled out as a cause of deficit.

Injuries where there is some degree of function below the level of the injury, be it motor or sensory, are classified as incomplete. The more function that remains the better the prognosis for recovery. Any sacral sparing (perianal sensation, voluntary rectal motor tone, flexion of the great toe) shows that there is at least partial continuity of the white matter long tracts and that the injury is incomplete. It is important to remember that sacral function might be the only deficit and must be both examined and documented.

It is possible to record the degree of injury according to the Frankel Classification (Frankel *et al*, 1969). This is as follows:

A: Absent motor and sensory function.

B: Sensory intact, absent motor function.
C: Sensory intact, motor function 2–3/5.
D: Sensory intact, motor function 4–5/5.
E: Sensory and motor function intact.

Conclusions

Injuries to the lumbar spine account for 15% of spinal injuries and may be associated with neurological disruption. It is vital to make a full, documented neurological examination of the lumbar-sacral nerve roots, including perianal sensation and anal tone in any trauma patient. Triple immobilisation on a long spinal board is essential until the spine can be cleared by physical examination and X-rays, particularly in the presence of any distracting injuries.

Key points

- Fifteen percent of spinal injuries occur in the lumbosacral region.
- Triple immobilisation on a spinal board during patient transfer will help minimise further injury.
- Initial assessment of all trauma patients should include assessment of the lumbar spine during initial 'log roll'.
- Neurological injuries caused by trauma to the spinal cord or cauda equina are possible complications.
- Early diagnosis is essential in optimising outcome.

References

Bolesta MJ *et al* (1996) Fracture and dislocation of the thoracolumbar spine. In: Rockwood, CA, Green DP *et al*, eds. *Fractures in Adults*. Lippincott-Raven, Philadelphia: 1529–71

Chance GQ (1948) Note on a type of flexion fracture of the spine. *Br J Radiol* **21**: 452–3

Denis F (1983) The three-column spine and its significance in the classification of acute thoraco-lumbar spinal injuries. *Spine* **8**: 817–31

Frankel HL, Hancock DO, Hyslop G *et al* (1969) The value of postural reduction in the initial management of closed injuries of the spine with paralegia and tetraplegia. *Paraplegia* **7**: 179–92

Krantz B, eds (1997) *Advanced Trauma and Life Support for Doctors*. American College of Surgeons, Chicago, IL: 217–53

CHAPTER 7

Pelvic fractures

Nicholas Wardle and Fares Haddad

Introduction

Pelvic fractures are associated with a high mortality and morbidity and their presence should be considered in all high energy traumas. Early management is directed towards Advanced Trauma Life Support (ATLS) principles but it is essential to be aware of the diagnosis and management of these complex injuries.

Anatomy

The pelvis transmits weight-bearing forces from the axial spine to the lower limbs and provides origin for muscles operating the hip, knee, spine, as well as abdominal and perineal muscles. It is formed by a bony ring consisting of the two innominate bones and the sacrum. The innominate bone is formed by the fusion of three ossification centres at the acetabulum: ilium, ischium and pubis. The innominate bones are joined anteriorly at the symphysis pubis and posteriorly to the sacrum at the sacroiliac (SI) joint.

The SI joint has two components, an articular portion – located anteriorly and comprising articular cartilage on the sacral side and fibrous cartilage on the ilium, and a fibrous portion – located posteriorly.

The pubic symphysis has hyaline cartilage on the medial (articular) aspect of the pubis. It is surrounded by fibrocartilage and a thick band of fibrous tissue.

There are strong ligaments contributing to the stability of the pelvic ring and these are outlined in *Table 7.1*.

Neural structures of important note are the sciatic nerve, which exits the pelvis deep to the piriformis; the lumbosacral trunk, which crosses the anterior sacral ala and SI joint; and the L5 nerve root, which exits below the L5 transverse process crossing the sacral ala.

Important vascular structures to remember are the internal iliac artery and its branches as these are of major importance in pelvic trauma. The notable anterior division branches are the inferior gluteal artery, which exits the pelvis via the greater sciatic notch; the internal pudendal artery, which is commonly injured in pelvic fractures; and the obturator artery, which may be disrupted in pubic rami fractures. The posterior division is more prone to damage as

Table 7.1. Ligaments of the pelvic ring

Ligament	Position	Comments
Posterior sacroiliac (SI) ligaments	(1) Short component run from posterior ridge of sacrum to posterosuperior and posteroinferior iliac spines (2) Long component run from lateral sacrum to posterosuperior iliac spines (and merges with sacrotuberous ligament)	Considered to be the strongest ligaments in the body
Anterior SI ligaments	From ilium to sacrum	
Sacrotuberous ligaments	From posterolateral sacrum and dorsal aspect of posterior iliac spine to ischial tuberosity	Along with posterior SI ligament it maintains vertical stability of pelvis
Sacrospinous ligaments	From lateral edge of sacrum and coccyx to sacro-tuberous ligament and inserts on ischial spine	Separates the greater and lesser sciatic notches
Iliolumbar ligaments	From L4 and L5 transverse processes to posterior iliac crest	Stabilises spine to pelvis
Lumbrosacral ligaments	From L5 transverse process to sacral ala	

a result of posterior pelvic displacement and it is the superior gluteal artery (the largest branch of the internal iliac artery supplying predominantly the gluteal muscles) that is the most commonly injured vessel in posterior pelvic disruptions. However, it is the pelvic veins (or, moreover, the massive venous plexus that drains into the internal iliac vein) that are the major source of haemorrhage in most pelvic fractures.

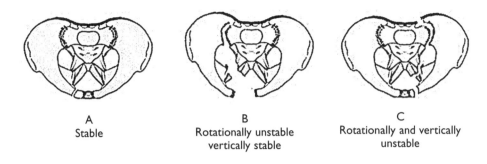

A	B	C
Stable	Rotationally unstable vertically stable	Rotationally and vertically unstable

Figure 7.1. Tile Classification (simplified).

The close proximity of the genitourinary system to the pelvis results in a high incidence of injuries, primarily to the bladder and urethra although vaginal injuries from bony spikes are not uncommon.

Mechanism of injury

Pelvic fractures are an important group of injuries and account for 1–3% of fractures. Sixty percent occur in men (Dalal *et al*, 1989). High-energy fractures that cause disruption to the pelvic ring are commonly caused by motor vehicle accidents, crush injuries, and falls from heights.

Clinical picture

High-energy pelvic ring fractures are often associated with severe or life-threatening soft tissue injuries. The mortality of pelvic ring fractures is in the region of 15–25% with open pelvic fracture carrying mortality in excess of 50%. Associated soft tissue injuries include vascular, genitourinary, abdominal, neurological and open fractures.

Early management of pelvic fractures is the management of the life-threatening associated injuries. This is a combination of assessment and treatment following ATLS guidelines.

Classification

Pelvic fractures have been classified by Tile (1988) based on the mechanism of injury into anteroposterior compression, lateral compression, or vertical shear fractures (*Figure 7.1*). Further classification by Burgess *et al* (1990) indicates the fracture patterns likely to be associated with major haemorrhage. These classifications are useful in the early management of pelvic ring fractures.

Management

Trauma team treatment is aimed at rapidly ensuring a patent airway and that breathing and circulation are established. Multiple large-bore intravenous lines are established allowing prompt restoration of circulation. Application of a pelvic belt may be required for early stabilisation of the circulation in patients with unstable pelvic fractures. Early recognition and appropriate initial treatment of all the soft tissue complications of pelvic ring fractures is important for overall outcome as inappropriate initial management may well prejudice the definitive surgical treatment of the pelvic fracture and its associated injuries.

Physical examination

Physical examination should include the following.

- Bimanual compression and distraction of the iliac wings – assesses for rotational instability.
- Manual leg traction – can aid in determining vertical instability.
- Rectal examination – a high riding prostate may indicate a urethral tear in males, the sacrum is palpated for irregularity.
- Vaginal examination – bleeding or lacerations indicate open fractures.
- Perineal skin – lacerations may indicate an open fracture (hyperabduction of the leg).

Radiographic evaluation

An anteroposterior view of the pelvis is obtained as part of the trauma series, this can identify up to 90% of pelvic injuries. Further radiographic views may be required to improve diagnosis and these include the pelvic inlet view (approximately 45° caudal tilt to show AP displacement), the pelvic outlet view (approximately 45° cephalad tilt to show superior-inferior displacement), lateral sacral view (identifies transverse sacral fractures), and computed tomography (CT), which offers the best visualisation of SI joints.

Associated injuries

Common associated major injuries involve the central nervous system, chest and abdomen. Haemorrhage occurs in 75% of patients with pelvic fractures; it is the leading cause of death and requires aggressive fluid resuscitation. There are three sources of bleeding: osseous, vascular and visceral. In up to 40% of patients there is an intra-abdominal source of bleeding. Arterial bleeding only occurs in 10–15% of patients. Bleeding from the pelvic venous plexus can result in a retroperitoneal haematoma of up to 4 litres in volume. Stabilising an unstable pelvic ring limits the pelvic volume and therefore the volume of haematoma that can form. The fastest method of achieving initial skeletal stability is by application of a pelvic belt that can stabilise both the anterior and posterior pelvic ring. Pelvic belts are only a temporary measure for controlling a pelvic fracture, and where application of a pelvic belt achieves haemodynamic control, a pelvic external fixator is often required.

Associated musculoskeletal injuries occur in 60–80% of patients, urogenital injuries being seen in 12%, and lumbosacral plexus injuries in 8%. The mortality rate is 15–25%.

Open pelvic fractures

Open pelvic fractures carry mortality in excess of 50%. There is potential for major vascular injury with haemorrhage and a high incidence of gastrointestinal and genitourinary injuries. A high proportion of these patients die at the scene of the accident or fail to respond to resuscitation. Overwhelming pelvic sepsis is the commonest cause of death in those surviving the initial resuscitation. Those that survive the initial phase require emergency surgery to stabilise the pelvis, with debridement and washout of the open wounds, and a diverting colostomy with a distal washout to protect the pelvis from further contamination. Open pelvic fractures require an aggressive multidisciplinary approach to treatment.

Beyond the 'trauma room'

Following the initial phase of emergency treatment and patient stabilisation, the definitive plan for fracture management is made. Stable type lateral compression fractures that do not cause significant disruption to one side of the pelvis allow patients to mobilise non-weight bearing until the fracture unites. Unstable fractures are those that are likely to go on to a malposition or non-union, cause pain, and neurological or other soft tissue complications if the patient mobilises. These unstable fractures may require operative stabilisation in order to allow effective nursing, to avoid prolonged bedrest and allow the patient to mobilise early. Deep vein thrombosis is very common following major pelvic fractures and may complicate operative treatment. The other main risks of operative treatment are infection, heterotopic ossification, delayed union and non-union. Operative treatment, if indicated, should be carried out by surgeons trained in pelvic reconstructive surgery and preferably in a tertiary referral pelvic unit.

Conclusion

A patient with a high energy injury should be examined carefully for the presence of a pelvic injury and emergency resuscitation commenced as soon as possible. Despite great effort there is still a high mortality rate from these injuries and subsequent morbidity may be long lasting.

Treatment of the pelvic fracture requires an understanding of local anatomy.

Repeated examination of an unstable pelvis disrupts early haemostasis and should be avoided. An experienced orthopaedic trauma surgeon should examine the pelvis as part of the trauma team management at an early stage, minimising secondary trauma from repeated examination before stabilising the fracture.

A multi-disciplinary team approach is required for the rehabilitation of these patients who often present with complex rehabilitation problems including chronic pain, neurological deficit, urological impairment, impotence, psychological disturbance, as well as reduced mobility.

Key points

- Pelvic fractures are caused by high energy injuries and are associated with other life-threatening injuries.
- There remains a significant mortality rate in patients presenting with pelvic fractures of up to 25%.
- Correction of hypovolaemia is essential and may require definitive surgical stabilisation.
- A simple 'pelvic belt' may prove life saving in a haemodynamically compromised patient.
- An experienced orthopaedic trauma surgeon should be involved in the case from the outset.
- Long-term morbidity from the pelvic fracture and associated injuries is a common problem.

References

Burgess AR, Eastridge BJ, Young JWR *et al* (1990). Pelvic ring disruptions: Effective classification system and treatment protocols. *J Trauma* **30(7)**: 848–56

Dalal SA, Burgess AR, Siegel JH *et al* (1989) Pelvic fractures in multiple trauma: Classification by mechanism is key to pattern of injury, resuscitative requirements and outcome. *J Trauma* **29**: 981

Raffa J, Christiensen NM (1976) Compound fractures of the pelvis. *Am J Surg* **132**: 282

Tile M (1988) Pelvic ring fractures: Should they be fixed? *JBJS* **70B**:1-12

Tile M (1996) Acute pelvic fractures. II. Principles of management. *J Am Acad Orthop Surg* **4(3)**: 152–61

CHAPTER 8

Injuries to the brachial plexus

Rahul Patel, Ken Mannan and Thomas Carlstedt

Introduction

There are two principal types of injury to the brachial plexus: the first is due to violent trauma and the second is sustained during birth. The former will be discussed in this chapter.

It is important to understand the anatomy of the brachial plexus, its reaction to injury and how to assess and treat these injuries, as they can be severely debilitating. It is well established that the best outcome follows early intervention. Brachial plexus injuries occur in 1.2% of polytrauma victims; motor vehicle accidents are the commonest cause, in particular, motorcycle accidents (Midha, 1997). Seventy percent of patients with brachial plexus lesions have associated injuries (Narakas, 1985).

Anatomy

The brachial plexus is formed from the fifth to eighth cervical and first thoracic spinal nerves (*Figure 8.1*). These spinal nerves combine into trunks in the posterior triangle of the neck.

- C5 and C6 combine to produce the upper trunk.
- C7 continues alone.
- C8 and T1 combine to produce the lower trunk.

These then divide behind the clavicle into anterior and posterior divisions:

- The three posterior divisions form the posterior cord.
- The lateral cord is formed by the anterior divisions of the upper and middle trunks.
- The medial cord is the direct continuation of the anterior division of the lower trunk.

Mechanism of injury

The mechanism of injury and the level of energy imparted are the most important

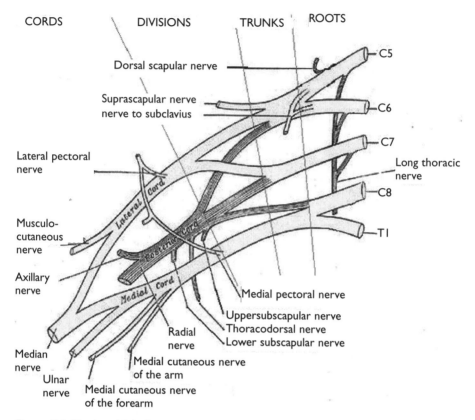

CORDS   DIVISIONS   TRUNKS   ROOTS

Dorsal scapular nerve

C5

Suprascapular nerve
nerve to subclavius

C6

Lateral pectoral
nerve

C7

Long thoracic
nerve

C8

Musculo-
cutaneous
nerve

T1

Axillary
nerve

Medial pectoral nerve

Uppersubscapular nerve
Thoracodorsal nerve
Lower subscapular nerve

Radial
nerve

Median
nerve

Medial cutaneous nerve
of the arm

Ulnar
nerve

Medial cutaneous nerve
of the forearm

Figure 8.1. The brachial plexus.

determinants of the degree of injury and prognosis (Birch *et al*, 1998). Open wounds, fractures, dislocations of the shoulder and vascular injury may occur near and be associated with brachial plexus injury.

Trauma, where the head and neck are violently deviated from one another, suggest severe injury and can cause multiple root avulsions from the spinal cord and ruptures of the spinal nerves (Barnes, 1949).

Roots are avulsed or ruptured. Rupture of the spinal nerves or trunks occurs frequently. The middle and upper trunks commonly rupture while the lower trunks (C8 and T1 spinal nerves) are usually avulsed from the spinal cord. The roots exit the vertebral foramina with diminishing downwards inclination such that roots C8 and T1 are almost at right angles to the cord and because there are no transverse radicular ligaments below C7, the lower roots are more susceptible to avulsion than the upper ones.

Injury to the lower roots can also result from being crushed between the first rib and clavicle.

Blunt trauma tends to result in lesions in continuity whereas penetrating lesions are likely to produce nerve lacerations.

Clinical picture and investigations

History and examination

Typically the patient presents with partial or complete loss of all or some part of upper limb motor function and concurrent diminished or absent sensation. Coupled with the mechanisms of injury highlighted above, this should alert the examining clinician to the possibility of brachial plexus injury.

History taking is critical and must include time of injury. Further contemporaneous documentation is paramount. The onset of symptoms must be elicited; acute single traumatic injury must be differentiated from progressive neurological deficit due to ongoing compressive insult. Local haematoma can cause delayed compression and ischaemia of the plexus in whole or in part. This is likely to be progressive and the paralysis and sensory abnormalities deepen with time.

The history of pain should include type and distribution as well as time of onset. Pain is usually associated with partial lesions (some fibres divided, others intact) or root avulsion injuries. Complete lesions are commonly painless. Symptoms change over time but resolution of pain does not indicate that recovery of function will ensue.

Sensory loss may not be complete in depth or distribution; it is likely to be altered and patchy. The latter suggests a non-degenerative or partial lesion (see below).

Motor function should be carefully recorded. One must be aware that associated injuries (fracture or dislocation) can make this difficult. Active and passive ranges of motion should be assessed. Individual muscles must then be examined with the aim of determining at which level the injury has occurred and which elements of the brachial plexus are involved.

For both sensory and motor assessment the Medical Research Council (MRC) grading systems should be used (*Tables 8.1* and *8.2*).

Detailed examination technique will not be discussed here but the following paradigms should be followed for a systematic approach: start proximally and work distally. Horner's syndrome should be looked for. Feel for upper limb pulses and auscultate for bruits. A Tinel's sign should be checked for; this can indicate a degenerative lesion as there is direct mechanical irritation of damaged axons (see below). However a negative Tinel's sign does not exclude a degenerative lesion.

An assessment of the autonomic system is mandatory. It can distinguish a non-degenerative lesion from a degenerative one. The smaller unmyelinated axons, transmitting deep pain and sympathetic function, are more resilient than large myelinated (light touch, proprioception, motor) axons to pressure or minor trauma. Thus the smaller axons are only lost if the fibres are cut (degenerative lesion). Changes in sweating, skin temperature and colour should be examined for.

Table 8.1. Medical Research Council grading for power

M0	Absence of contraction
M1	Visible muscle contraction, but no movement
M2	Muscle contraction and movement with gravity removed
M3	Muscle contraction able to overcome gravity
M4	Muscle contraction sufficient to offer resistance to active movement
M5	Normal

Table 8.2. Medical Research Council grading for sensation

S0	Absence of sensibility
S1	Deep cutaneous pain sensibility
S2	Some superficial cutaneous pain and tactile sensibility
S3	Some cutaneous pain and tactile sensibility without overreaction
S3+	S3 but with some two-point discrimination ability
S4	Normal

Finally, the arterial part of the neurovascular bundle can be injured at the same level as the plexus. The state of the peripheral circulation and swelling should be recorded. Rupture of the axillary vein produces oedema of the entire upper limb; rupture of the axillary artery may produce massive swelling of the upper limb and progressive rapid neurological deficit.

Investigations

Investigations should be tailored to the clinical findings. An X-ray of the cervical spine may reveal fracture or instability. A chest X-ray may show an elevated hemidiaphragm caused by phrenic nerve injury from a proximal avulsion injury to the upper parts of the plexus.

Magnetic resonance imaging (MRI) is useful for imaging cervical spine trauma and elucidating vascular injury. Brachial plexus injury can be identified by MRI, but referral to a specialist centre should not be delayed waiting for this investigation.

Angiogram is indicated in ischaemia complicating nerve injury. On-table angiography is extremely useful when undertaking vascular repair, but should not delay surgery.

Computed tomography (CT)-myelogram can confirm root avulsions; a pseudo meningocele indicates, but does not prove, root avulsion.

Nerve conduction studies (NCS) examine the electrical conductivity of large diameter, myelinated axons (sensory and motor). Root rupture can be pre-

or post-ganglionic. Sensory loss results if the lesion separates the dorsal root ganglion from the spinal cord (pre-ganglionic), but the axons do not degenerate as the cell body remains in contact with them. Lesions distal to the dorsal root ganglia (post-ganglionic) also cause loss of sensibility, but conduction is not detectable because the axons degenerate.

Electromyelography (EMG) measures the electrical activity within target muscles. Interpretation is broadly divided into spontaneous and voluntary. An intact nerve conveys stability to motor end plates and prevents spontaneous firing. Spontaneous activity, fibrillation or sharp waves indicate a degenerative injury to some or all axons supplying that muscle.

Nerve conduction studies and EMG are not useful before 7–10 days after injury because the distal part of the nerve does not die immediately and continues to conduct for several days (Chaudhry and Comblath, 1992). Following a degenerative lesion a motor response to stimulation distally can last for 3–4 days and the electrical response can continue for a further 6–7 days.

Some EMG information may be relevant at two weeks but the nature of the lesion takes up to six weeks to manifest. Nerve conduction studies and EMG after six weeks can give a good indication of prognosis.

Classification

Nerve injury produces two types of lesion: degenerative and non-degenerative. Interruption of the connection between the cell body and the axon leads to Wallerian degeneration, with disintegration and death of the nerve fibres distal to the injury and consequently conduction stops. This may occur from division of the nerve and its integument (neuronotmesis) or from disruption of the axons only (axonotmesis). Non-degenerative lesions display conduction block of varying severity but retained nerve cell structure. This type of injury can deepen to become axonotmesis (ie. a degenerative lesion) if the insult producing this condition is prolonged or increased.

Lesions to the brachial plexus can be supra-, retro- or infra-clavicular (*Figure 8.2*). Double level lesions can occur in 15% of cases.

Management

Initial management

The patient with multiple injuries or involved in high-energy trauma must be assessed and resuscitated according to the Advanced Trauma Life Support (ATLS) guidelines. Limb threatening vascular injuries should be addressed within the first two hours of injury, immediately after stabilisation of life-threatening conditions.

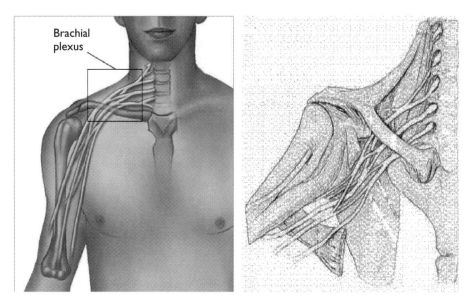

Figure 8.2. Relationship of the brachial plexus to the clavicle.

In assessment of nerve injury, the most important consideration after vascularity is not to assume that the injury is due to conduction block. This can be said only if there is preservation of deep pain and sympathetic function. Non-degenerative lesions will progress to degenerative ones if there is ongoing insult (eg. expanding haematoma, aneurysm, displaced fracture/dislocation) even if conduction block is present.

Progressive neurological deficit indicates ongoing insult and requires urgent exploration for decompression. Dislocations and severely angulated fractures should be reduced as soon as possible.

An injury to the brachial plexus should be dealt with promptly. Early referral to local or on-site expertise must be made within hours of injury. Direct repair, nerve grafting, nerve transfer or decompression might be carried out. Recent studies using molecular biology have shown the importance in timing of nerve repair. One month after injury, the expression of growth factors and their receptors declines to the extent that outcome of repair is less favourable than if done immediately after injury (Gordon *et al*, 2003). Time-dependent neuron death adds urgency to the reconstruction of root avulsion injuries as replanting the avulsed ventral root to some extent maintains the population of spinal cord motoneurons (Carlstedt *et al*, 1993).

Definitive management

Nerve grafts for repair are usually taken from the same limb so that further deficit does not occur. The medial cutaneous nerve of the forearm or the superficial radial nerves are commonly used. Nerve transfers include spinal accessory nerve to the suprascapular nerve to restore shoulder stability. Ulnar nerve fasicles can be transferred to the biceps muscle to restore elbow flexion.

There are limited late nerve and tendon transfers available to the most seriously injured patients. Neuropathic pain can be debilitating. Intercostal nerve transfers can alleviate pain. Pharmacological approaches involve the standard analgesic ladder, incorporating muscle relaxants and membrane-stabilising agents. The anti-epileptic medications gabapentin, pregabalin and carbamazepine have been used with some success in modulating pain.

Conclusion

Brachial plexus injury is usually associated with high-energy trauma and particular mechanisms of injury. The incidence of concomitant musculoskeletal and vascular injury is not uncommon. Systematic assessment according to ATLS principles initially and careful examination of the upper limb subsequently will reveal the level of injury and the type of lesion to the plexus. Prompt referral to local expertise is paramount in treating these injuries as the outcome of surgery is more favourable if performed early. The sequelae of brachial plexus injury can be debilitating and a multidisciplinary approach is often needed.

Key points

- Violent trauma to the upper body can result in brachial plexus injury. The complete loss of movements in the arm and shoulder with loss of sensation with a Horner's sign and no Tinel sign when tapping the posterior triangle of the neck indicates the most severe injuries to the brachial plexus (avulsion of C5 through T1).
- An understanding of the anatomy will aid examination and diagnosis.
- Associated vascular and musculoskeletal injuries are common. These must be examined for and treated urgently as ongoing insult from local injury can 'deepen' lesions.
- Contemporaneous documentation is necessary throughout. The use of MRC grading systems is recommended.
- Prompt referral to local expertise for surgery is advised as early intervention yields the best outcome.
- Although imaging investigations are useful (MRI, CT, angiography), waiting for these must not delay referral.
- Nerve conduction studies are not helpful before 7–10 days after injury. Electromyography is most useful after six weeks, when coupled with nerve conduction studies, as indicators of prognosis.

References

Barnes R (1949) Traction injuries of the brachial plexus. *J Bone Joint Surg* **31B**: 10–16

Birch R, Bonney G, Wynn-Parry CB, eds (1998) *Surgical Disorders of the Peripheral Nerves.* London: Churchill Livingstone: 123–55

Carlstedt T, Hallin RG, Hedstrom KG, Nilsson-Remahl IA. (1993) Functional recovery in primates with brachial plexus injury after spinal cord implantation of avulsed ventral roots. *J Neurosurg Psychiatry* **56**: 649–54

Chaudhry V, Comblath DR (1992) Wallerian degeneration in human nerves: Serial electrophysiological studies. *Muscle Nerve* **15**: 687–93

Gordon T, Sulaiman O, Boyd JG (2003) Experimental strategies to promote functional recovery after peripheral nerve injuries. *J Peripheral Nerv Syst* **8**: 236–50

Midha R (1997) Epidemiology of brachial plexus injuries in a multi-trauma population. *Neurosurgery* **40**: 1182–9

Narakas AO (1985) The treatment of brachial plexus injuries. *Int Orthop* 9: 29–36

CHAPTER 9

Common injuries of the shoulder

Simon Jennings and Brian Cohen

Introduction

Shoulder injuries may occur by direct impact, eg. as the result of high-energy collisions as in a road traffic accident or sport, or indirectly where the force is transmitted via the arm to the shoulder complex, eg. a fall onto an outstretched hand. Standard assessment begins by taking a history of the injury and fully examining the patient. Imaging should relate to clinical findings.

Shoulder (glenohumeral) dislocation

The shoulder joint has low intrinsic stability from its osseous structure. It relies on soft tissue for stability, specifically the glenoid labrum, capsular ligaments and the rotator cuff. Dislocation usually involves significant trauma or congenital laxity (or both). Of dislocations 95% are anterior, and only 5% are posterior. Inferior dislocation may occur (luxatio erecta) but this is very rare.

Clinical picture

The shoulder classically dislocates anteriorly in the position of apprehension: abduction and external rotation. Posterior dislocations occur after direct trauma or muscle spasm and are associated with epilepsy, alcohol and electrocution.

A patient with an anterior dislocation characteristically presents with the arm slightly abducted and in internal rotation. The shoulder will lose its normal deltoid contour, appearing 'squared'. The humeral head may be palpated anteriorly. In posterior dislocation the arm is held adducted and internally rotated. The shoulder may appear flat anteriorly and will not externally rotate. In luxatio erecta the arm is held abducted ('statue of liberty'). The neurovascular status of the arm must be assessed and recorded before and after any attempt at reduction.

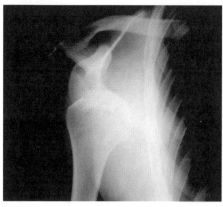
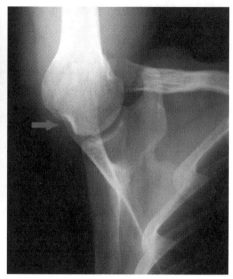

Figure 9.1. (above) Anterior dislocation
– anteroposterior view.
Figure 9.2. (right) Hill–Sachs lesion of
humeral head.

Investigations

Standard radiographs should be taken to confirm the direction of dislocation and the presence of any concomitant fracture (glenoid, greater or lesser tuberosity). An anteroposterior (AP) view in the plane of the scapula will show most anterior dislocations with the humeral head displaced medially and the joint surface no longer aligned with the glenoid. A Stryker notch view may show an impaction fracture (Hill–Sachs lesion) of the posterolateral aspect of the humeral head (*Figures 9.1* and *9.2*).

Posterior dislocations are less common and may be missed on AP radiograph as the humeral head appears aligned with the glenoid; the key to diagnosis is the shape of the humeral head – the 'light-bulb' or 'drumstick' sign. Posterior dislocation of the shoulder is more easily diagnosed on axillary or lateral scapular views.

Management

Any dislocation should be reduced as soon as possible. Delay may make reduction harder and may increase damage to other structures. Before reduction neurovascular examination should be carried out to define any existing deficit. The axillary nerve, which supplies the deltoid and is sensory to the skin in the 'shoulder patch' region, is at risk in dislocation as it is closely related to the glenohumeral joint. Sensation and active abduction should be tested and recorded before reduction. Vascular injuries occur very rarely but are more common in elderly patients and are probably related to the relatively stiff vessel walls.

Most dislocations can be reduced by closed means. Ideally reduction should be with full relaxation under a general anaesthetic but this is not normally possible. Reduction is therefore carried out in an appropriately equipped setting with adequate sedation and analgesia. A number of recognised, well-described techniques can be used to reduce the shoulder (see *Further reading*).

Posterior dislocations are reduced by traction of the arm in adduction (forceful external rotation may cause fracture). Inferior dislocations can usually be reduced by traction alone – occasionally the humeral head buttonholes the capsule and requires open reduction.

Surgical exploration and open reduction is indicated if there is an associated vascular injury, an open dislocation, failed closed reduction, a displaced fracture of glenoid or greater tuberosity, and in persistent instability after reduction.

Post-reduction management requires re-evaluation of neurovascular status and repeat X-ray. Most surgeons immobilise the shoulder for 3–6 weeks, but there is no evidence that prolonged immobilisation reduces the incidence of recurrent dislocation. Early mobilisation is encouraged in patients over 40 years to prevent stiffness. Posterior dislocations may be unstable after reduction and may require special bracing or immobilisation of the shoulder in a plaster of Paris spica.

The main complications of dislocation include recurrent dislocation, neurological injury, fracture and associated rotator cuff tear or vascular injury. The risk of recurrent dislocation is inversely related to the age at first dislocation. In patients under 20 years up to 80% have a recurrent dislocation in the next 2 years. After the age of 40 years there is a 10–15% redislocation rate. Rotator cuff tears are more common in older patients with dislocation (up to 60% in patients over 50 years of age). This will delay healing and rehabilitation. If function is impaired then early repair is indicated.

Shoulder (glenohumeral) fracture-dislocation

Fractures of the tuberosities are seen in older people. Anterior dislocation is associated with a fracture of the greater tuberosity and posterior dislocation with a fracture of the lesser tuberosity. After reduction of the dislocated joint the fracture is often reduced but a post-reduction X-ray is important to ascertain this.

Open reduction and internal fixation may be required if the fragment remains significantly displaced (*Figure 9.3*).

Fractures of the scapula

Fractures of the scapula are rare, constituting 3–5% of all shoulder injuries. There is a high likelihood of other serious injury. Initial assessment should treat any life-

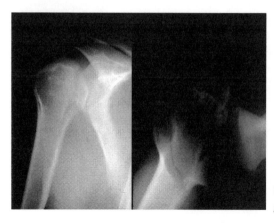

Figure 9.3. Anterior dislocation with greater tuberosity fracture.

threatening condition first following the Advanced Trauma Life Support (ATLS) protocols. Once medically stabilised the shoulder can be assessed.

Clinical picture

Trauma may be direct or indirect through the outstretched arm. The patient presents with pain, especially on active and passive shoulder movement and on deep inspiration. There may be local tenderness to palpation, swelling, ecchymosis and deformity. Full neurovascular examination is required.

Investigations

Scapula fractures are diagnosed on plain X-rays. Subsequent information can be gained from specific scapular views. Computed tomography (CT) scans with three-dimensional reconstruction are helpful in evaluating the need for surgical intervention.

Management

Most scapula fractures are treated non-operatively. Glenoid fossa fractures are rare, comprising 10% of scapula fractures. These can result in glenoid incongruity and instability and may have a poor outcome if treated non-operatively.

Glenoid neck fractures do not involve the joint surface and tend to heal in their position of displacement. Open surgical reduction may be required if the position is likely to interfere with rotator cuff function (angulation >40°, displacement >1cm). Fractures of the clavicle in association with glenoid fractures, may constitute a 'floating shoulder', so both fractures should be fixed as they will tend to displace with time.

Coracoid fractures commonly occur at the base and are typically minimally displaced. These can be managed conservatively in most instances.

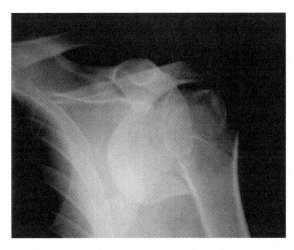

Figure 9.4. Three part fracture of neck of humerus.

Fractures of the scapula body will usually not require any intervention but there is a high incidence of other major injury in these patients.

Fracture of proximal humerus

Fracture of the proximal humerus in the young patient is a high-energy injury, while in the elderly with osteoporosis the fracture is more commonly a result of a low-energy fall.

Clinical picture

The patient will present with a history of injury to the shoulder. There will be pain and a decreased range of motion. The shoulder may have an abnormal alignment if the shaft is displaced or angulated. Initial assessment must include neurovascular assessment. Distal pulses may be present even in the presence of vascular injury.

Investigation

Radiographs of the shoulder are essential to plan treatment. These should include AP, scapular lateral and axillary views. Occasionally these may need to be supplemented with rotated views to see the tuberosities (*Figure 9.4*).

Management

Proximal humeral fractures are classified and management is planned according to whether the head, greater tuberosity or lesser tuberosity are involved and their degree of displacement (Neer, 1975). Most fractures are minimally displaced and can be managed conservatively with immobilisation followed by early range of motion exercise. Displaced fractures may require either closed reduction or open reduction and internal fixation. Severely displaced four-part fractures, involving both tuberosities and the surgical neck, require primary hemiarthroplasty.

Neurovascular complications may occur. The brachial plexus and axillary artery are at risk from injury by the humeral shaft, which is nearby.

Conclusion

Injuries to the shoulder are commonly encountered in the emergency department. Accurate assessment and timely initial management is required. Early identification of those patients who will require surgical intervention will help to optimise outcome.

Key points

■ Patients presenting with glenohumeral dislocation must have axillary nerve function documented prior to and following manipulation
■ Fractures of the scapula are associated with high energy trauma and their presence should raise clinical suspicion of associated injuries.
■ Displaced proximal humeral fractures may require surgical intervention and orthopaedic input should be sought at an early stage

---

Reference

Neer CS II (1975) Four segment classification of displaced proximal humerus fractures. *Am Acad Ortho Surg Instructional Course Lectures* **24**: 160–8

Further reading

Barton N, Mulligan P (1999) *The Upper Limb and Hand.* Saunders, London

Dee R, Hurst LC, Gruber MA, Kottmeier SA (1997) *Principles of Orthopaedic Practice.* 2nd edn. Blackwell Science, Oxford

Rowe CR (1956) Prognosis in dislocation of the shoulder. *J Bone Joint Surg* 38-A: 951–77

CHAPTER 10

Injuries to the clavicle and acromioclavicular joint

Sam Oussedik

Anatomy and function

The clavicle is a doubly curved long bone (*Figure 10.1*) that acts as the only osseous strut connecting the trunk to the shoulder and arm. Medially the clavicle articulates with the manubrium of the sternum at the sternoclavicular joint, while laterally it articulates with the acromion of the scapula at the acromioclavicular joint. Trapezius and deltoid muscles attach to the flat outer third, as do the acromioclavicular and corococlavicular ligaments. The tubular medial third is a boundary of the cervicoaxillary canal, and as such affords protection to the neurovascular bundle supplying the upper limb, including the brachial plexus, subclavean and axillary vessels. The junction between these two different cross-sectional configurations occurs in the middle third, which constitutes an area vulnerable to injury.

The acromioclavicular (AC) joint is also vulnerable to injury. Its horizontal stability is maintained by the AC ligaments, while its vertical stability is maintained by the corococlavicular (CC) ligaments.

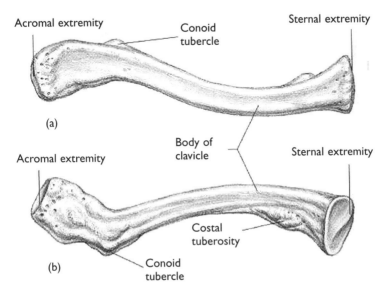

Figure 10.1. Anterior (a) and posterior (b) views of the clavicle.

Mechanisms of injury

It is a commonly held belief that the majority of clavicle fractures result from a fall onto the outstretched hand. However, the commonest mechanism is in fact a fall onto the shoulder, accounting for some 87% of injuries; direct impact on to the clavicle leads to 7%, and a fall onto the outstretched hand is responsible for the remaining 6% (Stanley *et al*, 1988).

Following fracture, the sternocleidomastoid (SCM) muscle elevates the medial fragment, while the weight of the upper limb leads to a depression of the lateral fragment.

Injuries to the AC joint follow similar mechanisms. A fall onto the shoulder with the arm in adduction leads to the acromion being driven medially and inferiorly. A fall onto the outstretched hand can also lead to AC joint disruption.

Clinical presentation

The patient with a clavicle fracture usually presents with the ipsilateral arm splinted in adduction across the chest, its weight supported by the contralateral arm, thus unloading the injured clavicle. As described above, the clavicle plays an important role in protecting the neurovascular structures of the upper limb as they traverse the cervicoaxillary canal. Thus clinical examination must include a careful neurovascular assessment of the affected upper limb, comparing with the contralateral side. The integrity of the skin over the clavicle should be assessed. As the medial fragment is elevated by the action of SCM it often leads to tenting of the overlying skin (*Figure 10.2* and *Figure 10.3*).

Associated injuries which should be excluded include:

- ipsilateral pneumothorax following apical lung injury
- head injury
- cervical spine injury
- acromioclavicular injuries
- sternoclavicular injuries
- scapulothoracic injuries
- rib injuries.

Radiographic examination should include an anteroposterior view and a 45° caudal tilt view. These usually suffice to show injury to the proximal and middle thirds. However, these views tend to overexpose the distal third. If an injury to the distal third is suspected, then anterior and posterior 45° oblique views centred over the distal clavicle should be obtained. If injury to the ligamentous

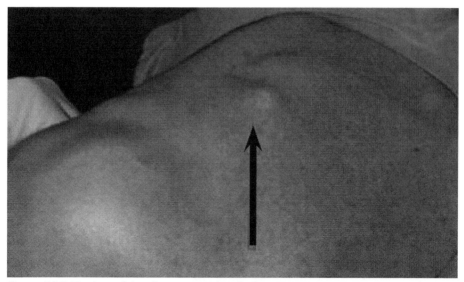

Figure 10.2. Tenting of the skin over a clavicle fracture.

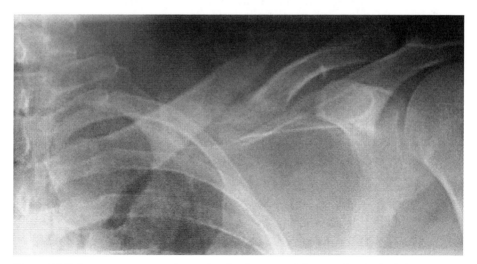

Figure 10.3. Anteroposterior radiograph of a fracture of the middle third of the clavicle.

structures of the AC joint are suspected, then stress views can be obtained, with the patient having a 10-pound weight strapped to the ipsilateral wrist.

Injuries to the AC joint may present in a similar fashion. Examination of the patient in a sitting position with the affected arm dependant will help to accentuate any deformity. A 'step-off' of the injured AC joint may be noted, with possible tenting of the skin over the distal clavicle. Tenderness is often elicited over the injured joint, together with a reduced range of motion of the affected shoulder, limited by discomfort. Once again, associated injuries should be excluded.

Radiographic examination with standard shoulder views (anteroposterior, scapular-Y and axillary) often suffices. Further examination of the ligamentous structures can be obtained through stress radiography, obtained in a similar fashion to that described above.

Classification of injuries

Clavicle fractures are commonly classified according to anatomical description:

* open vs. closed injuries
* location – proximal, middle or distal thirds
* displacement
* angulation
* pattern – transverse, oblique, spiral, greenstick
* comminution.

In addition, the Allman classification can be used (Allman, 1967). This groups fractures according to their anatomical site, with subgroups according to the fracture pattern.

* Group I: Fractures of the middle third
* Group II: Fractures of the distal third
  * Type 1: Minimal displacement
  * Type 2: Fracture medial to the corococlavicular ligaments
  * Type 3: Intra-articular fractures
* Group III: Fractures of the medial third
  * Type 1: Minimal displacement
  * Type 2: Displaced
  * Type 3: Intra-articular
  * Type 4: Epiphyseal separation
  * Type 5: Comminuted

Disruption of the AC joint is classified according to the displacement of the distal clavicle, and the associated ligamentous disruption (*Figure 10.4*). A type I injury results from a force applied to the shoulder insufficient to disrupt either AC or CC ligaments. This represents an AC ligament strain. Type II injuries result from a tear to the AC ligaments while the CC ligaments remain intact. A separation is seen between the distal clavicle and the acromion. Type III and IV injuries result from complete disruption of both AC and CC ligaments, with displacement of the distal clavicle superiorly or posteriorly. Type V shows greater superior displacement of the distal clavicle, resulting from additional disruption of the muscular attachments. Type VI occurs when the distal clavicle

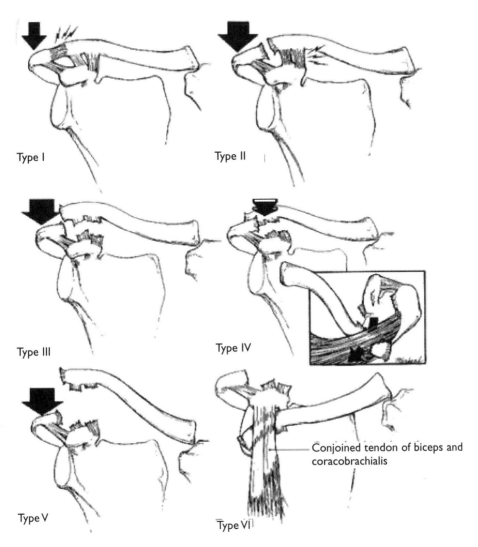

Figure 10.4. Rockwood classification of ligamentous injuries to the AC joint (From Rockwood et al, 1996).

is displaced inferiorly to the coracoid process and posteriorly to the biceps and coracobrachialis tendons.

Management

Non-operative treatment is appropriate for the majority of clavicle fractures. Comfort and pain relief are the main treatment goals, with the arm held in a broad-arm sling for 4–6 weeks. The overall prevalence of non-union at 24 weeks after the fracture in non-operatively treated clavicle fractures has been found to be 6.2%, with 8.3% of the medial end fractures, 4.5% of diaphyseal fractures, and 11.5% of lateral end fractures remaining ununited (Robinson *et al*, 2004).

Operative treatment should be considered in the following cases:

- Open fractures.
- Associated neurovascular injuries.
- Gross displacement of the fracture with tenting of the skin.

Management of AC joint disruption depends on the pattern of injury according to the classification system shown above.

- Type I: Non-operative management, provision of a broad-arm sling and adequate analgesics. Rest for 7–10 days and refrain from full activity until a painless full range of motion is restored.
- Type II: Non-operative management, provision of a broad-arm sling and adequate analgesics. Gentle range of motion exercises should be commenced as soon as possible, with a return to full activities at around 6 weeks.
- Type III: Treatment for these injuries is controversial. Schlegel (2001) reports reasonable results for non-operative treatment at 1 year. However, operative management may be necessary in the treatment of heavy labourers and young active patients in order to ensure an earlier return to full activity.
- Type IV: Operative treatment by open reduction and surgical repair of the CC ligaments for vertical stability.
- Type V: Operative treatment by open reduction and surgical repair of the CC ligaments for vertical stability.
- Type VI: Operative treatment by open reduction and surgical repair of the CC ligaments for vertical stability.

Operative management

Operative treatment of clavicle fractures involves open reduction and internal fixation, usually by a combination of plate and screws (*Figures 10.5* and *10.6*).

Operative management of acromioclavicular joint disruption involves open reduction of the displaced distal clavicle and stabilisation of the AC joint. This can be accomplished by the Weaver-Dunn procedure, as illustrated in *Figure 10.7*.

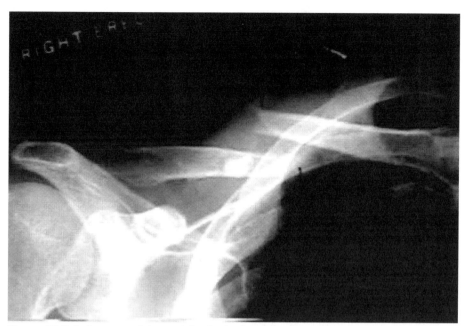

Figure 10.5. A fracture of the middle third of the clavicle, with superiorly displaced medial fragment endangering the overlying skin.

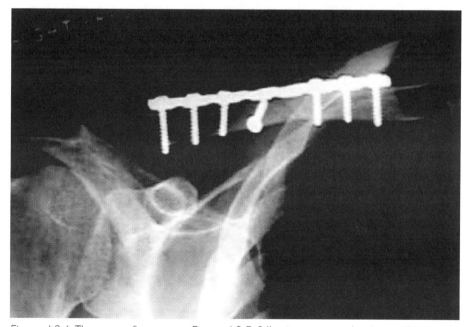

Figure 10.6. The same fracture as Figure 10.5 following open reduction and internal fixation.

The Weaver-Dunn procedure

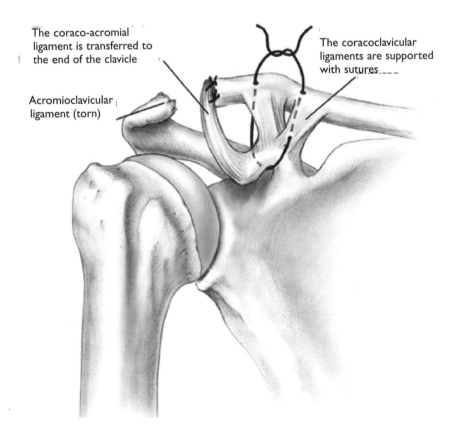

The coraco-acromial
ligament is transferred to
the end of the clavicle

The coracoclavicular
ligaments are supported
with sutures

Acromioclavicular
ligament (torn)

Figure 10.7. The Weaver-Dunn procedure for the treatment of chronic AC joint disruption (Weaver and Dunn, 1972).

Key points

- Clavicle fractures commonly result from a fall onto the affected shoulder.
- The vast majority can be treated non-operatively.
- Accurate classification of acromioclavicular joint injuries allows early intervention in those requiring operative management

References

Allman FL Jr (1967) Fractures and ligamentous injuries of the clavicle and its articulation. *J Bone Joint Surg Am* **49**: 774–84

Robinson CM, Court-Brown CM, McQueen MM, Wakefield AE (2004) Estimating the risk of nonunion following nonoperative treatment of a clavicular fracture. *J Bone Joint Surg Am* **86**: 1359–65

Rockwood CA Jr, Green DP, Bucholz RW, Heckman JD (eds) (1996) *Rockwood and Green's Fractures in Adults*. 4th Edn. Vol. 2. Philadelphia: Lippincott-Raven: 1354

Schlegel TF (2001) A prospective evaluation of untreated acute Grade III acromioclavicular separations. *Am J of Sports Med* **29**: 699–703

Stanley D, Trowbridge EA, Norris SH (1988) The mechanism of clavicular fracture. A clinical and biomechanical analysis. *J Bone Joint Surg Br* **70(3)**:461–4

Weaver JK, Dunn HK (1972) Treatment of acromioclavicular injuries, especially complete acromioclavicular separations. *J Bone Joint Surg Am* **54**: 1187

CHAPTER 11

Injuries of the humerus

Claire Young

Anatomy

The humeral shaft is triangular in cross-section and runs from just proximal to the insertion of pectoralis major to the metaphyseal flare and supracondylar ridge distally. It is the long bone of the arm connecting the shoulder to the elbow joint.

The midshaft of the humerus has a notable groove posteriorly, the spiral groove. This is the landmark for the course of the radial nerve traversing from the medial to the lateral side of the humerus. The nerve is tethered as it emerges from the groove and pierces the intermuscular septum. It is at this point that it is most prone to injury in humeral shaft fractures (*Figure 11.1*).

Mechanism of injury

Fractures to the humeral shaft constitute about 1% of all fractures. They occur either as a result of direct blows, which lead to transverse or short oblique fractures with or without a butterfly fragment, or as a result of a fall on the outstretched hand with a twisting injury which causes a spiral fracture.

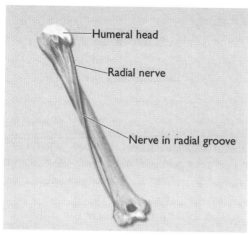

Figure 11.1. Humerus showing course of radial nerve in spiral groove.

Clinical picture

Patients present with a history of trauma, pain in the affected limb, swelling and inability to use the limb, and may or may not have an obvious clinical deformity depending on the degree of injury to the soft tissues overlying the bone in the affected individual.

Clinical evaluation of the patient, after taking an appropriate history, should involve assessment of the whole limb. The brachial, radial and ulnar pulses should be

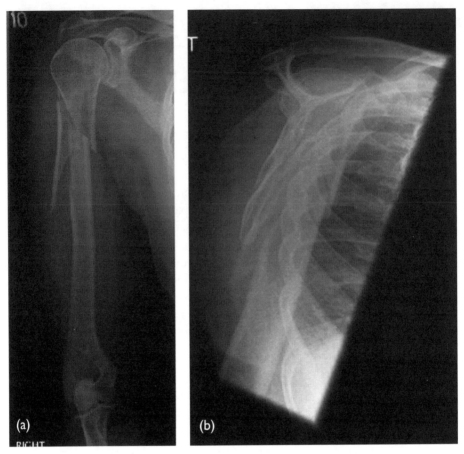

Figure 11.2. (a) Anteroposterior and (b) lateral radiographs of spiral comminuted fracture of the right proximal humerus.

evaluated. The functional status of all the nerves should be assessed, most especially the radial nerve.

Radial nerve injuries

Injuries to the radial nerve occur in 18% of humeral shaft fractures. This is usually either a middle third fracture or a Holstein–Lewis fracture (an oblique fracture of the distal third). The radial nerve supplies the muscles to the extensor compartment of the forearm. Evaluation of the nerve's function includes the patient's ability to extend the wrist (extensor carpi radialis longus, extensor carpi radialis brevis, and extensor carpi ulnaris), extend the fingers (extensor digitorum communis, extensor indicis proprius) and extend the thumb (extensor pollicis longus). The sensory distribution of the radial nerve is the skin of the first dorsal web space of the hand.

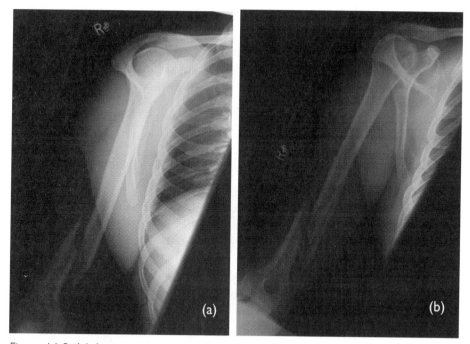

Figure 11.3. (a) Anteroposterior and (b) lateral radiographs of spiral fracture of the right distal humerus.

Injury can either be laceration of the nerve by the fracture fragments, entrapment of the nerve in the fracture site or a traction injury causing a neuropraxia. About 90% of radial nerve palsies following a humeral shaft fracture recover in 3–4 months. Nerve conduction studies and electromyography can be performed at 4–6 weeks to assess nerve recovery.

Both anteroposterior and lateral radiographs of the humerus should be requested, with the shoulder and elbow joint included on each (*Figures 11.2* and *11.3*).

Classification

Humeral shaft fractures are classified descriptively:

- open or closed
- position in shaft (proximal, middle or distal third)
- transverse, oblique, spiral, segmental
- butterfly fragment or comminution
- angular, translational or rotational deformity or shortening.

Knowledge of the muscle attachments to the humerus can help in the understanding of the main deforming forces following fractures at different levels. In fractures above the level of the pectoralis major insertion the proximal fragment tends to abduct and internally rotate because of the pull of the rotator cuff muscles, while the distal shaft is displaced medially and anteriorly by pectoralis major. In fractures below the deltoid insertion the proximal fragment is abducted and pulled forward by deltoid and coracobrachials while the distal fragment is drawn upward. These fractures are commonly displaced and over-ride.

Management

Initial

If the fracture is open then it should be treated as any open injury with intravenous antibiotics, surgical debridement of the wound and fracture stabilisation.

Closed injuries require fracture reduction and immobilisation. When the fracture is undisplaced the arm can be immobilised with a U slab (a moulded plaster slab around the medial and lateral aspects of the arm from the shoulder to the elbow). For displaced fractures the application of a hanging cast will help to correct angular deformities.

A hanging cast is useful in fractures that occur distal to the deltoid insertion as it can help in fracture reduction, as described by Caldwell in 1940. It involves using the weight of the forearm in association with a lightweight cast to act as traction to bring about fracture reduction. A lightweight cast is applied from approximately 3cm proximal to the fracture site to the wrist with the elbow at 90° and the forearm in neutral. A plaster loop is applied at the wrist on the radial border of the forearm to support the sling. The patient should not support the elbow in any way and he/she should sleep upright to maintain the traction force on the fracture. Positioning of the sling loop is important to correct angular deformities at the fracture site.

Once the cast is applied check radiographs are taken. If there is lateral angulation at the fracture site then the loop should be placed on the dorsum of the wrist, if there is medial angulation the loop should be positioned on the volar aspect of the wrist. The rotation of the forearm then allows the angular deformity to be corrected. The length of the sling is also critical. If the sling is too long, allowing the forearm to drop below the horizontal, then the distal fragment will tilt posteriorly leading to anterior angulation at the fracture site. If the sling is too short then the reverse occurs, giving posterior angulation of the fracture. Hanging casts are useful in the initial treatment and reduction of displaced oblique or spiral fractures. If used for transverse fractures they tend to distract the fragments and lead to a non-union.

Definitive

Humeral shaft fracture treatment is conservative with a union rate of over 90%.

Table 11.1. Operative indications for diaphyseal fractures of humerus

Open fractures	Association with vascular injuries
Segmental fractures	Floating elbow
Pathological fractures	Polytrauma
Failure of conservative management	Radial nerve dysfunction following fracture manipulation

Functional braces are the most common method of fracture immobilisation, either initially or following fracture reduction in a hanging cast for a couple of weeks (Sarmiento *et al*, 1977). This is a functional orthosis, which brings about fracture reduction by compression of the soft tissue envelope, allowing for elbow and shoulder movement.

Some malalignment of humeral fractures can be accepted without compromising function or cosmetic appearance: 10–20° of anterior angulation, 10–30° of varus and 2cm shortening do not compromise the limb function because of the wide range of movement that is possible at the shoulder (Klenerman, 1969).

Operative intervention is indicated in some circumstances (*Table 11.1*). Options are open reduction and internal plate fixation, intramedullary nailing or external fixation (*Figure 11.4*).

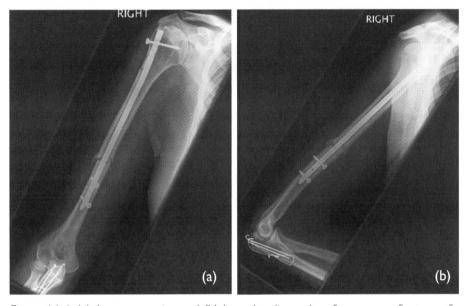

Figure 11.4. (a) Anteroposterior and (b) lateral radiographs of transverse fracture of the right humerus following intramedullary nailing.

Key points

■ Humeral shaft fractures are common injuries.

■ Careful evaluation of radial nerve function, both sensory and motor, is required in all patients who sustain humeral shaft fractures.

■ The treatment of closed humeral shaft fractures is non-operative.

References

Caldwell JA (1940) Treatment of fracture of the shaft of the humerus by hanging cast. *Surg Gynecol Obstet* **70**: 421

Klenerman L (1969) Experimental fractures of the adult humerus. *Med Biol Eng* **7**: 357

Sarmiento A, Kinman PB, Galvin EG, Schmitt RH, Phillips JG (1977) Functional bracing of fractures of the shaft of the humerus. *J Bone Joint Surg* **59A**: 596–601

CHAPTER 12

Injuries around the elbow

A Reza Jenabzadeh and Fares Haddad

Introduction

The elbow joint is a complex hinge that is important for the range of motion and mobility of the upper limbs. Injuries of the elbow fall into two groups: those of children (supracondylar fractures, medial and lateral condylar fractures, fractured neck of radius, pulled elbow) and those of adults (fractured distal humerus, radial head fractures, olecranon fractures, elbow dislocations).

The elbow is second only to the distal forearm for frequency of fractures in children. Boys are injured more often than girls and more than half the patients are under 10 years old. Elbow fractures in adults pose a different problem from those in children. Fusion in the epiphyses alters the mechanical properties, and consequently leads to differences in the pattern of injury. This chapter offers an overview of common elbow injuries.

Clinical anatomy

The elbow joint consists of articulation between the humerus, radius and ulna. The extra-articular medial and lateral epicondyles of the distal humerus are separated by the intra-articular trochlea and capitellum. The trochlea articulates with the proximal ulna and the capitellum articulates with the radial head. The distal humerus is angled anteriorly at about 30°. The distal articular surface of the humerus is angulated 7° of valgus to the long axis. This, combined with the ulnar angulation of the olecranon, give a carrying angle of 20° with the elbow in full extension.

There are four muscle groups responsible for muscle movement: the extensors, consisting of triceps brachii and anconeus, and the flexors, comprising brachialis, biceps and brachioradialis. Forearm supination is performed by biceps and supinator, and forearm pronation is performed by pronator teres and pronator quadratus.

The medial collateral ligament consists of two slips and originates from the medial epicondyle.The anterior slip inserts into the coronoid process and the posterior slip inserts into the olecranon The lateral collateral ligament originates from the lateral epicondyle and inserts onto the annular ligament and the olecranon. The annular ligament surrounds the radial neck and stabilises the radioulnar articulation.

Table 12.1. CRITOE mnemonic highlighting age at which ossification centres appear

Centre	Age
Capitellum	2 years
Radial head	4 years
Internal (medial) epicondyle	6 years
Trochlea	8 years
Olecranon	10 years
External (lateral) epicondyle	12 years

The normal elbow has an extension-to-flexion arc up to 145°. Normal pronation and suppination are about 80° and 85°, respectively. Function arcs for activities of daily living require 50° pronation and suppination and 100° arc of extension to flexion between 30° and 100°.

X-ray interpretation of the bony anatomy also has its problems in children. This is because the bone ends are largely cartilaginous and therefore radiographically incompletely visualised. The secondary ossification centres can be seen on X-ray and should not be mistaken for fracture fragments. The mnemonic CRITOE helps remember the ages at which ossification centres appear (*Table 12.1*).

Variations occur and if there is any difficulty in interpreting the radiographs, films of the other side should be taken for comparison.

Mechanism of injury

Elbow injuries generally result from direct trauma to the elbow or a fall on an outstretched hand.

Clinical findings and investigations

Patients with elbow injuries generally present complaining of pain resulting in restricted movement at the joint. They usually hold the elbow flexed supported by the uninjured arm and are very reluctant to be examined. Depending on the severity of the injury bruising and swelling may be visible if there is no obvious deformity. All bony prominences (olecranon, radial head, medial and lateral epicondyles) should be palpated to see if they elicit any pain. An attempt should be made to assess the range of movement in the elbow and any level of ligament laxity. This is usually aided by infiltration of the elbow joint with some local anaesthetic.

Neurovascular injuries around the elbow joint should not be forgotten. Distal pulses and any motor/sensory deficit should be checked with all elbow injuries.

Elbow injuries in children

Supracondylar fractures

Supracondylar fractures are the most common elbow injuries, occuring in 60% of cases. The fracture line lies just proximal to the trochlea and capitellum. The distal fragment may be displaced posteriorly (hyperextension injury; 95% of all cases) or anteriorly (flexion injury; rare). There is tenderness, swelling and deformity over the distal humerus, and the child generally resists examination.

Supracondylar fractures can be classified according to severity of displacement (Wilkins, 1984). Type I is an undisplaced fracture. Type IIa is a greenstick fracture with posterior tilting of the distal fragment. Type IIb is a more severe greenstick fracture with both angulation and malrotation. Type III is a completely displaced fracture.

Type I fractures are immobilised in a cast. Type IIa can be reduced under general anaesthetic with the arm then held in a collar and cuff. Type IIb and III fractures should be reduced under general anaesthetic and held by percutaneous wires. If this fails, open reduction and internal fixation is required.

Medial and lateral condylar fractures

Medial and lateral condylar fractures account for less than 5% of all distal humeral fractures. The lateral side is more commonly fractured than the medial side. The child (generally 3–4 years of age) falls on the hand with the elbow extended and forced into varus or valgus. The child usually presents with a swollen painful elbow, and a loss of the normal carrying angle.

Milch (1964) classified these fractures into two groups for both medial (*Figure 12.1*) and lateral (*Figure 12.2*) epicondylar fractures. The lateral trochlear ridge is the key to classifying trochlear fractures.

In type I fractures, the lateral trochlear ridge remains intact, with the intact condyle providing medial to lateral elbow stability. In type II fractures, the lateral trochlear ridge is part of the fractured condyle. This is a less stable fracture as it may allow for radioulnar translocation if capsuloligamentous disruption occurs on the contralateral side.

The aim of treatment is the restoration of articular congruity to maintain normal elbow motion and to reduce the risk of post-traumatic arthritis. This is done nonoperatively for non- or minimally displaced fractures. Operative

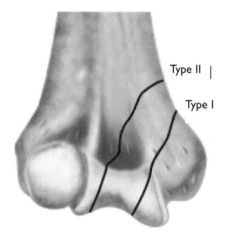

Figure 12.1. Medial condylar fractures.

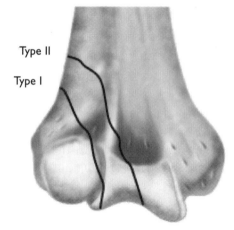

Figure 12.2. Lateral condylar fractures.

treatment is reserved for open or displaced fractures. This consists of screw fixation and/or collateral ligament repair if necessary.

Fractured neck of radius

Following a fall the child complains of pain in the elbow. There may be tenderness over the radial head and pain on rotating the forearm. In children, up to 30° of radial head tilt and up to 3mm of transverse displacement are acceptable. Beyond this, reduction is required, either by closed manipulation or open reduction, and internal fixation is unnecessary.

Pulled elbow

This injury is seen in children between the ages of 2–6 years. There is a usually a clear history of a traumatic incident involving traction of the arm (eg. parent suddenly pulls on a child's hand to prevent him or her from running out onto a road). The radial head stretches and slips out from under cover of the annular ligament. The child is fretful and refuses to move the joint.

Reduction can easily be achieved by:

- Placing the wrist in full radial deviation and forcibly supinating the arm.
- Rapidly pronating and supinating the forearm.

If these measures fail, the arm should be rested in a sling when spontaneous reduction usually occurs within 48 hours.

Elbow injuries in adults

Fractures of the distal humerus

Three types of distal humeral fractures have been described (Muller *et al*, 1991):

- Type A is an extra-articular supracondylar fracture. These are rare fractures that usually require open reduction and internal fixation.
- Type B is an intra-articular unicondylar fracture.
- Type C includes bicondylar fractures with varying degrees of comminution.

Intra-articular fractures (types B and C) are high-energy injuries. Sometimes the fracture extends into the metaphysic as a T- or Y-shaped break.

Undisplaced fractures can be treated with a posterior slab with the elbow at 90°. Open reduction and internal fixation is the treatment of choice for displaced type B and C fractures

Fractured capitellum

This articular injury occurs when the patient falls on an outstretched hand. The anterior part of the capitellum is sheared off and displaced proximally. Undisplaced fractures are treated by simple splintage. Displaced fractures are openly fixed with a small screw or, if this proves too difficult, the fragment is excised.

Fractured head of radius

This injury is caused by a fall on the outstretched hand. The radial head impacts against the capitellum. There is well-localised tenderness over the radial head and pain on pronation and supination. Four types of fracture are identified (Mason, 1954) (*Figure 12.3*). Type I is a vertical split in the radial head. Type II has a single fragment of the head broken off and displaced. Type III is a comminuted fracture. Type IV is a radial head fracture with an elbow dislocation.

Type I fractures can be treated non-operatively. Type II should have the fragment reduced and held with a small screw. In type III fractures attempts should be made to reconstruct the radial head, but if this is not possible it should be excised and replaced with a silicone or metal prosthesis. Type IV is the same as management of type III with relocation of the joint.

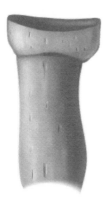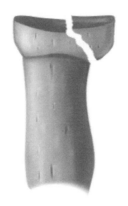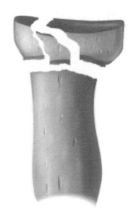

Figure 12.3. Mason classification of radial head fractures.

Olecranon fracture

Two types of injury are seen:

- A comminuted fracture as a result of direct trauma.
- A clean transverse break, as a result of traction when the patient falls onto the hand while the triceps muscle is contracted.

Clinically the patient may still be able to extend the elbow against gravity. Displaced fractures (2mm) are an indication for operative treatment with tension-band wiring.

Elbow dislocation

Elbow dislocation accounts for 12–28% of elbow injuries, seen at all ages. In 90% of cases the radioulnar complex is displaced posterolaterally. The patient supports his/her forearm with the elbow in slight flexion with obvious deformity, pain and swelling.

In uncomplicated dislocations the elbow can be manipulated back to position under sedation and analgesia. Surgery is indicated for cases of soft tissue and/or bony entrapment in which closed reduction is not possible. Dislocations may be complicated by associated fractures (eg. coronoid process, medial and lateral epicondyles and radial head) and these should be carefully looked for.

Key points

- Mechanism of injury is usually a fall on an outstretched hand or directly onto the point of the elbow.
- The aim of treatment is to try and get an anatomical reduction with as good a functional range of movement as soon as possible.
- A careful neurovascular examination is crucial and must be documented at presentation and after manipulation or reduction.
- Complications must be remembered. These include: stiffness, neurovascular injury, compartment syndrome leading to Volkmann's ischaemic contracture, growth disturbances, myositis ossificans, post-traumatic arthritis and non-union.

References

Mason ML (1954) Some observations on fractures of the head of the radius with a review of 100 cases. *Br J Surg* **42**: 123–32

Milch H (1964) Fractures and fracture dislocation of the humeral condyles. *J Trauma* **4**: 592–607

Muller ME, Allgower M, Schneider R *et al* (1991) *Manual of Internal Fixation*. 3rd edn. Springer Verlag, Berlin, Heidelberg, New York

Wilkins KE (1984) Fractures and dislocations in the elbow region. In: Rockwood CA Jr, Wilkins KE, King RE, eds. *Fractures in Children*. vol 3. JB Lippincott and Co, Philadelphia

CHAPTER 13

Forearm fractures

Rahul Patel and Fares Haddad

Introduction

The forearm serves an important role in upper extremity function, facilitating positioning of the hand in space. The movements of pronation and supination are universally integral in the activities of daily living. If function is to be restored following fracture, clear decisive management is required. The fractures of the shaft of either the radius, ulna or both are discussed in this chapter.

Anatomy and function

The forearm contains two bones, the radius and ulna.

The radius is the lateral bone in the forearm. Its upper end articulates with the humerus at the elbow joint and with the ulna in the superior radioulnar joint. Its lower end articulates with the scaphoid and lunate bones of the carpus at the wrist joint and the ulna at the inferior radioulnar joint. It has a sharp interosseous border medially for the attachment of the interosseous membrane that binds the radius and ulna together.

The ulna is the medial bone of the forearm. Its articulations are with the elbow and the radius above as described, and the radius inferiorly.

The forearm is enclosed in a sheath of deep fascia which is attached to the periosteum of the posterior subcutaneous border of the ulna. The fascial sheath, together with the interosseous membrane and fibrous intermuscular septa, divide the forearm into anterior and posterior compartments (*Figure 13.1*).

The anterior compartment contains the deep and superficial flexor muscles, the radial and ulnar arteries, superficial radial nerve, ulnar nerve, median nerve and their branches.

The posterior compartment contains the extensor muscles, the posterior interosseous nerve and artery (distally joined by the anterior interosseous artery).

The main movements of the forearm are pronation (0–95°) and supination (0–85°). These movements are only possible due the unique anatomy of the bones and the interosseous membrane, annular ligament, radioulnar ligaments and the triangular fibrocartilage complex at the wrist, binding them together, giving the bones the features of a linked parallelogram.

It is important to bear in mind the attachment of certain muscles (eg. pronator

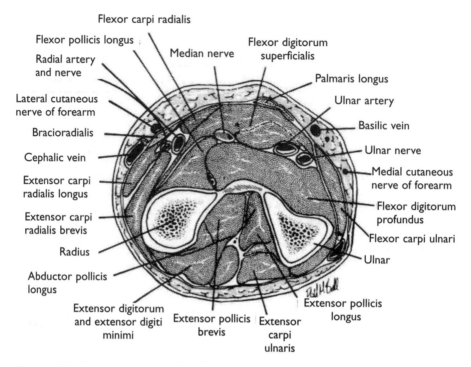

Flexor carpi radialis

Flexor pollicis longus

Radial artery and nerve

Lateral cutaneous nerve of forearm

Bracioradialis

Cephalic vein

Extensor carpi radialis longus

Extensor carpi radialis brevis

Radius

Abductor pollicis longus

Median nerve

Flexor digitorum superficialis

Palmaris longus

Ulnar artery

Basilic vein

Ulnar nerve

Medial cutaneous nerve of forearm

Flexor digitorum profundus

Flexor carpi ulnari

Ulnar

Extensor digitorum and extensor digiti minimi

Extensor pollicis brevis

Extensor carpi ulnaris

Extensor pollicis longus

Figure 13.1. Compartments of the forearm.

teres) and the normal appearance of the bones on standard anteroposterior (AP) and lateral radiographs.

Mechanisms of injury

Direct violence

Either of the forearm bones may be fractured, especially the ulna when, in a fall, the shaft strikes a sharp edge, or in self-defence when the forearm is used as a shield for the head and the shaft is struck with a hard object (night-stick injury).

Indirect violence

More commonly the forearm is injured in a fall onto the back or front of an outstretched hand. The force of impact on the hand stresses the forearm bones; commonly both bones fracture (*Figure 13.2*).

Fracture dislocations

If one forearm bone is seen to be fractured and angulated, it has inevitably

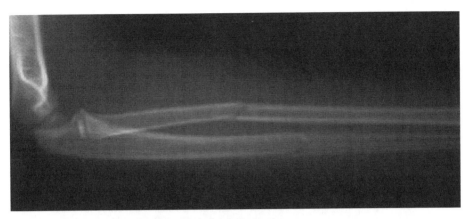

Figure 13.2. Fracture of both bones of the forearm.

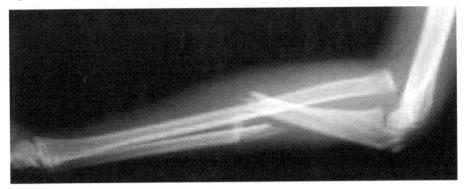

Figure 13.3. Monteggia fracture.

become relatively shorter. If its attachments to the wrist and humerus are intact, the other forearm bone must be dislocated. The commonest type of fracture-dislocation of this type is a fracture of the ulna with dislocation of the radial head – Monteggia fracture (Rang, 1968) (*Figure 13.3*).

The same pattern of injury occurs in the Galeazzi (Galeazzi, 1934; Rang, 1968) fracture-dislocation (*Figure 13.4*); here a dislocation of the distal ulna accompanies a radial shaft fracture. One should never accept fracture of a single forearm bone as an entity.

Axial rotation

When the radius fractures, contrary to the ulna, in addition to angulation one fragment may rotate relative to the other. A discrepancy in widths of the fragments at fracture level illustrates the presence of axial rotation. Pronator quadratus tends to pronate the distal fragment in all radial shaft fractures. In all proximal third radius fractures, pronator teres helps to pronate the distal fragment assisting pronator quadratus. The proximal fragment in this situation

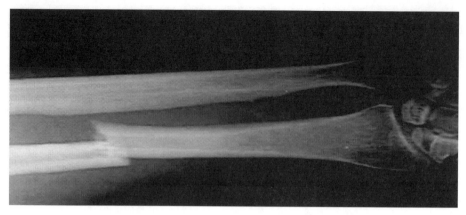

Figure 13.4. Galeazzi fracture

is fully supinated by biceps. In fractures of the distal third, biceps is opposed so the proximal fragment tends to lie in the mid (neutral) position. Axial rotation of the ulna is rare. One should check that in the lateral radiograph, olecranon, coronoid process and styloid process should all be visible.

Greenstick fractures

In children any intact periosteum on the original concave surface of the fracture exerts a constant force which may cause angulation if the plaster slackens (*Figure 13.5*). Reduction of these fractures requires manipulation only in the majority of cases. If there is offending, then shortening and instability are more likely and the reduction is more difficult.

Clinical picture and investigations

Deformity, pain, swelling and loss of function are the commonest presenting complaints in association with one of the mechanisms described above. History and examination are just as important as in any other medical scenario. The examination must assess and document neurovascular status of the affected limb. Take note of whether the injury is open or closed and treat accordingly with antibiotics and appropriate dressings if open.

Non-displaced fractures of both bones are rare. If the forearm is swollen and tense, a compartment syndrome must be excluded. In the obtunded patient, compartment pressures are mandatory.

Radiographs must include the elbow and wrist joint and two views (AP and lateral) must be obtained. Angulation, shortening and comminution should be noted and the proximal and distal radioulnar joints should be carefully assessed for the presence or absence of subluxation or dislocation. A line drawn through the radial shaft, head and neck should pass through the

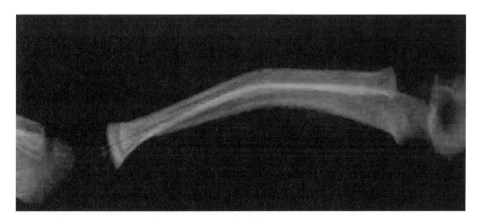

Figure 13.5. Greenstick fracture radius and ulna

centre of the capitellum on any view of the elbow. See *Figures 13.2* to *13.5* for radiographs of common fractures.

Classification

Fractures of both bones of the forearm are usually classified according to level of fracture, pattern of the fracture, degree of displacement, presence or absence of comminution or segmental bone loss and whether they are open or closed. For descriptive purpose it is useful to divide the forearm into thirds based on the linear dimensions of the radius and ulna.

Fractures of the radius alone are divided into two groups:

▪ Fractures in the proximal two-thirds of the bone not associated with injury to the distal radioulnar joint.
▪ Fractures at the junction of the middle and distal thirds that are associated with injury to the distal radioulnar joint (Galeazzi fracture).

Fractures of the proximal two-thirds of the radius are frequently associated with fracture of the ulna.

Isolated fractures of the ulna that are angulated more than 10° in any plane or displaced more than 50% of the diaphyseal diameter are classified as displaced. They can be associated with radial head instability (Monteggia fracture, the original description of which was anterior dislocation of the radial head). Bado (1967) described four distinct variations: types I and II are fractures of the ulna diaphysis at any level with anterior and posterior angulation, respectively, and anterior and posterolateral radial head dislocation, respectively. Type III is a fracture of the ulna metaphysic with lateral or anterolateral dislocation of the radial head while type IV is a fracture of the proximal third of the ulna and radius with anterior dislocation of the radial head.

Management

Initial

Following history, examination, and assessment of X-rays, if there is angulation and displacement or shortening of a single bone fracture, or fracture of both bones with or without rotation and angulation, referral to the orthopaedic team must be made. Analgesia must be given. Reduction must not be attempted in the accident and emergency setting. If an open injury has occurred it is best to allow the orthopaedic surgeon to see the open wound before immobilisation is applied.

Above elbow back-slab plaster of Paris is the most appropriate form of immobilisation for these types of fractures in patients of all ages. Isolated ulna fractures can be immobilised in a below elbow cast but if in doubt, apply an above elbow plaster. Non-compliant children may be placed in a broad-arm sling, having discussed this with the orthopaedic surgeon and provided definitive treatment will take place in the near future. Elevation, neurovascular observations and regular analgesia form the mainstay of initial management after stabilisation.

Definitive

Single bone greenstick fractures and the majority of radius and ulna fractures in children can be managed by manipulation under anaesthetic and a well-moulded cast. Only occasionally in severely displaced and unstable fractures is fixation required. In adults, non-displaced ulna shaft fractures can be treated conservatively although non-union and delayed-union are recognised complications. Both-bone fractures with minmal displacement and angulation may be manipulated and assessed for stability in theatre; stable fractures may be treated in plaster alone. Monteggia, Galeazzi, or both-bone displaced, shortened or rotated fractures often require open reduction and internal fixation. The radius is often reduced and fixed first. If dislocation of the radial head has occurred this may relocate closed but occasionally requires open reduction; radioulnar joint dislocation may need stabilisation with K-wires (*Figure 13.6*).

Cast application is paramount in all cases. The distal fragment (distal forearm) must be orientated to match the proximal; therefore in adult proximal radius fractures, the distal forearm must be supinated to match the proximal fragment as biceps brachii is the major deforming force. The more distal the fracture the more towards neutral rotation the distal fragment (forearm) may be placed to align the fracture. In children, posterior angulation should be placed in full supination and anterior angulated fractures in full pronation. Six to eight weeks in plaster is normally adequate especially if internal fixation has been performed. Longer periods may be needed in the elderly and shorter periods (4 –6 weeks) for children with greenstick type fractures. This is often followed

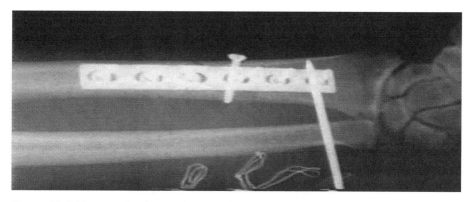

Figure 13.6. Plating of radius and K-wire fixation of diastasis of distal radio ulnar joint for Galeazzi fracture.

by a period of physiotherapy and rehabilitation which may take several months depending on the severity of the initial injury.

Conclusion

The correct management of forearm fractures is paramount if permanent loss of function is to be avoided. Knowledge of local anatomy and appreciation of associated injuries of the fracture facilitate correct investigations and obviate long-term morbidity. If there is any doubt in management, referral to the orthopaedic team is advised.

Key points

- The forearm is divided into two compartments: anterior and posterior.
- The main movements of the forearm are pronation and supination.
- It is important to bear in mind the attachment of certain muscles and the normal appearance of the bones on standard AP and lateral radiographs.
- Mechanisms of injury include direct violence (commonly the ulna), indirect violence, fracture dislocation (Monteggia and Galeazzi fractures), axial rotation (mainly the radius) and greenstick fractures in children.
- History and examination are just as important as in any other medical scenario. The examination must assess and document neurovascular status of the affected limb and note whether the fracture is open or closed.
- Radiographs must include the elbow and wrist joint and two views (AP and lateral) must be obtained.
- Referral to the orthopaedic team must be made if there is angulation and displacement or shortening of a single bone fracture, or fracture of both bones with or without rotation and angulation.

References

Bado JL (1967) The Monteggia lesion. *Clin Orthop* **50**: 70–86

Galeazzi R (1934) Uber ein Besonderes Syndrom bei Verltzunger im Bereich der Unterarmknochen. *Arch Orthop Unfallchir* **35**: 557–62

Rang M (1968) *Anthology of Orthopaedics*. E & S Livingstone, Edinburgh

CHAPTER 14

Injuries to the distal radius

Sam Oussedik

Anatomy

The distal radius includes the metaphysis, formed mainly of cancellous bone, supporting the articular surface (*Figure 14.1*). This articular surface is biconcave, allowing articulation with the proximal carpal row (the radio-carpal joint) and has a sigmoid notch for articulation with the distal ulna (the distal radio-ulnar joint).

The radius supports 80% of axial load, the remaining 20% being supported by the ulna and triangular fibrocartilage complex. This force transmission is dependent on the normal anatomical relationships of the radiocarpal joint and distal radio-ulnar joint (DRUJ) remaining intact.

The distal radius is the site of insertion of numerous ligaments. These often remain intact following fracture, aiding reduction through ligamentotaxis. Of the numerous neurovascular structures that traverse this region to supply the hand, particular attention should be paid to the median nerve when assessing injuries to the distal radius.

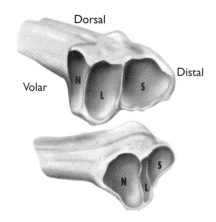

Figure 14.1. Anatomy of the distal radius. N: sigmoid notch; L: lunate articular surface; S: scaphoid articular surface.

Mechanisms of injury

The commonest mechanism of injury to the distal radius is a fall onto the outstretched hand, with the wrist between 40° and 90° of dorsiflexion. Axial force applied to the wrist in this position initially leads to the volar aspect of the distal radius failing in tension. As the fracture propagates, the dorsal aspect is compressed, leading to dorsal comminution. Impaction of the cancellous metaphysis leads to further dorsal instability, with the addition of shearing forces often leading to articular surface

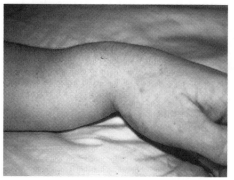

involvement. This type of low-energy fracture should be distinguished from high-energy injuries, such as those resulting from road traffic accidents, which can lead to significantly displaced, highly comminuted and highly unstable fractures.

Clinical picture and investigations

Figure 14.2. (left) Dinner fork deformity of the distal radius.

Typically patients present with pain localised to the distal forearm and wrist together with deformity. The nature of the deformity will depend on the displacement of the fracture. With dorsal angulation, the typical 'dinner fork' deformity is seen (*Figure 14.2*). The wrist will be swollen, with bruising, tenderness and a painful range of motion.

Clinical examination should include a careful neurovascular assessment. Radial and ulnar pulses should be palpated. Ulnar, radial and median nerves should be examined thoroughly, paying particular care to the median nerve. This travels through the carpal tunnel to supply motor innervation to the muscles of the thenar eminence and sensory fibres to the lateral three and a half digits. It is vulnerable to injury at this point through traction at the time of injury, direct trauma from fracture fragments, or increase in local pressure through haematoma formation or oedema. Symptoms of entrapment include paraesthesia in the thumb, index and middle fingers, and evidence of this should be sought in both history and examination.

The initial assessment should include examination of the ipsilateral elbow and shoulder to rule out associated injuries. Any suspicion should be investigated through the requesting of appropriate radiographs.

Initial radiographic assessment should include anteroposterior (AP) and lateral views of the wrist. Radiographs should be examined for:

- Articular involvement – requesting oblique views may help in assessing radiocarpal involvement.
- Radial shortening – measured on the AP view (*Figure 14.3*).
- Radial angulation – measured on the lateral view (*Figure 14.4*).
- Radial inclination – measured on the lateral view (*Figure 14.5*).
- Comminution.
- Stability – the tendency of the fracture to redisplace following reduction.

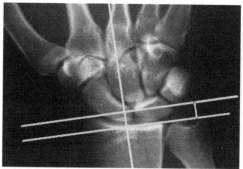

Figure 14.3. Radial length: two lines are drawn perpendicular to the long axis of the radius. The first line intersects the tip of the radial styloid and the second intersects the distal articular surface of the ulnar head. The distance between the two lines, the radial length, should be 11–12mm.

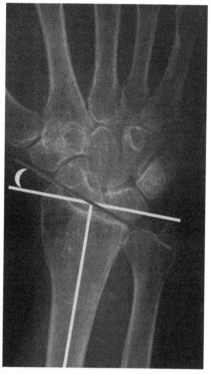

Figure 14.5. Radial inclination: one line is drawn from the tip of the radial styloid to the ulnar corner of the articular surface, and one line is drawn perpendicular to the long axis of the radius. Average radial inclination is 16°–23°.

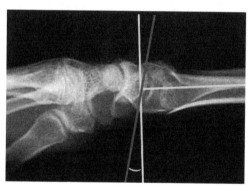

Figure 14.4. Volar tilt: one line is drawn perpendicular to the long axis of the radius, and one line is drawn along the articular surface. Normal volar tilt measures between 0° and 22° (mean 11°–14.5°).

Stable fractures tend to be extra-articular with mild to moderate displacement.

These measurements help to assess the deformity caused by any fracture, and plan for reduction if indicated. The most important factor governing outcome following treatment is the amount of articular depression, with any step-off greater than 2mm leading to a poorer outcome and an increased probability of post-traumatic osteoarthritis (Knirk and Jupiter, 1986).

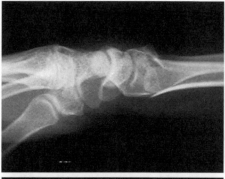
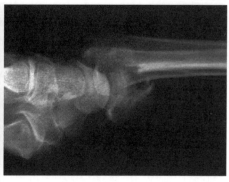
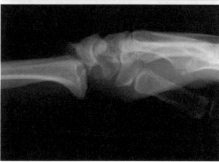

Figure 14.6. (above left) A Colles' type fracture showing dorsal angulation of the distal radial fragment.
Figure 14.7. (above right) A Smith's fracture with volar angulation of the distal radial fragment.
Figure 14.8. (left) A Barton's fracture showing dorsal subluxation of the radiocarpal joint.

Classification

Accurate classification aids communication between clinicians, and the application of the correct classification system allows accurate assessment of the injury.

Descriptive classification of the injury is often adequate and preferable to inaccurate use of classification systems. When describing the injury, the following should be noted:

- open vs closed
- displacement
- angulation
- comminution
- loss of radial length
- articular involvement.

Several eponyms are associated with distal radial injuries. Colles first described distal radial fracture following low-energy trauma occurring in the elderly population. A Colles' fracture is now accepted as being a low-energy injury in osteopenic bone, occurring in the over 50-year-old population. The fracture typically shows a combination of dorsal angulation (*Figure 14.6*), dorsal displacement, radial shift and radial shortening. While

Table 14.1. Frykman's classification of Colles' fractures

Type	Radius	Ulna	Radiocarpal	Radioulnar
I	Extra-articular	Absent	Absent	Absent
II	Extra-articular	Present	Absent	Absent
III	Intra-articular	Absent	Present	Absent
IV	Intra-articular	Present	Present	Absent
V	Intra-articular	Absent	Absent	Present
VI	Intra-articular	Present	Absent	Present
VII	Intra-articular	Absent	Present	Present
VIII	Intra-articular	Present	Present	Present

From Frykman (1967)

initially applied exclusively to extra-articular injuries, this term is now extended to intra-articular injuries as well. The Frykman classification (*Table 14.1*) subdivides this type of fracture according to whether the ulna styloid is avulsed, and whether the radiocarpal, distal radioulnar or both joints are involved.

A Smith's fracture (*Figure 14.7*) describes injuries with volar angulation of the distal radial fragment.

A Barton's fracture (*Figure 14.8*) is a fracture-dislocation, or subluxation of the radiocarpal joint. A rim of the distal radius remains associated to the carpus and displaces with it. Volar angulation is more common than dorsal, and both types are usually unstable, requiring operative treatment to maintain adequate reduction.

Management

Initial management

Having fully assessed the injury, together with patient factors such as age, hand dominance, occupation and level of physical activity, a decision must be made as to the appropriate management. The goal should be to provide the patient with the most comfortable and functional wrist possible.

Stable, minimally displaced fractures may be amenable to closed reduction and immobilisation in a cast. A number of anaesthetic options are available:

- Local anaesthetic via a haematoma block.
- Regional anaesthesia via a Bier's block.
- Sedation and analgesia.

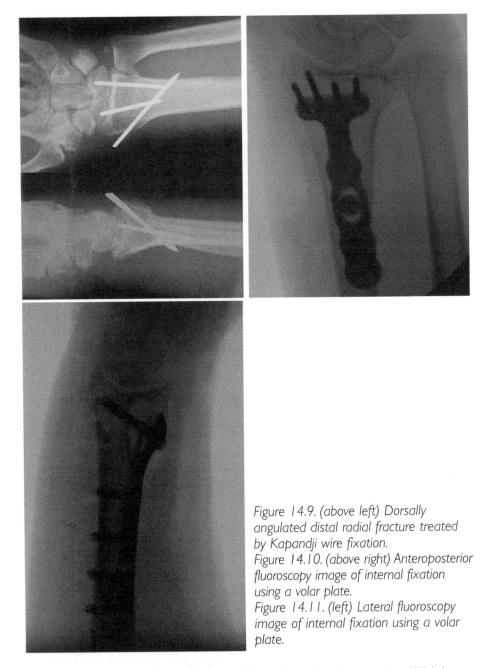

Figure 14.9. (above left) Dorsally angulated distal radial fracture treated by Kapandji wire fixation.
Figure 14.10. (above right) Anteroposterior fluoroscopy image of internal fixation using a volar plate.
Figure 14.11. (left) Lateral fluoroscopy image of internal fixation using a volar plate.

The choice of method will depend largely on local protocols. Whichever method is selected, it should ensure the ability to manipulate the fracture with a minimum of discomfort, allowing maintenance of reduction while a cast is applied.

Adequate reduction is achieved when the deformity is reversed to within normal limits, assessing the post-reduction radiograph in a similar manner to the initial film. A neurovascular examination should follow manipulation, once again paying particular attention to the median nerve. Persistent symptoms should warrant consideration for operative decompression of the carpal tunnel. All patients should be reviewed at regular intervals, with initial review at one week, to confirm maintenance of adequate reduction.

Operative management is reserved for those patients with fractures that are unstable or in which adequate reduction cannot be achieved through closed methods.

Definitive management

The choice of appropriate operative management is governed by the pattern of injury. A number of procedures are available to the surgeon, including:

- External fixation – bridging and non-bridging devices.
- Closed reduction and percutaneous wiring.
- Open reduction and internal fixation – with or without bone grafting.

Unstable extra-articular fractures can be treated by closed reduction guided by fluoroscopy, and fixation through percutaneous wires. The Kapandji technique (Kapandji, 1987) is often used in the treatment of dorsally angulated fractures (*Figure 14.9*). Here, two wires are passed through the fracture site itself and used to lever the dorsally angulated fragment into the correct position.

Volar angulation and comminution is more difficult to control with percutaneous techniques, and open reduction and internal fixation are often required to gain and maintain adequate reduction (*Figures 14.10* and *14.11*).

Conclusions

Fractures to the distal radius are a common injury seen in the accident and emergency department. It is important to differentiate between low-energy fractures in osteopenic bone seen in older patients and high-energy injuries in younger patient groups. Accurate assessment of articular involvement and deformity is vital in deciding on appropriate management. Manipulation under sedation or local or regional anaesthesia followed by immobilisation in an appropriate cast will suffice for the majority of extra-articular injuries. Intra-articular injuries, especially in younger patients, will often require operative treatment.

Key points

■ Injuries to the distal radius are commonly encountered in the accident and emergency department.

■ Accurately assessing displacement of the involved fragments will aid selection of appropriate treatment.

■ Treatment should be aimed at maximising comfort and function.

■ Extra-articular, dorsally angulated fractures may well be treated by closed manipulation and immobilisation in a plaster cast.

■ Other types of fractures may require operative management.

References

Frykman G (1967) Fracture of the distal radius including sequelae-shoulder-hand-finger syndrome, disturbance in the distal radio-ulnar joint and impairment of nerve function. A clinical and experimental study. *Acta Orthop Scand Suppl* **108**: 3

Kapandji A (1987) Internal fixation by double intrafocal pinning. Functional treatment of non articular fractures of the lower end of the radius. *Ann Chir Main* **6**: 57–63

Knirk JL, Jupiter JB (1986) Intra-articular fractures of the distal end of the radius in young adults. *J Bone Joint Surg* **68A**: 647–59

CHAPTER 15

Injuries of the carpus and scaphoid

Rahul Patel and Fares Haddad

Introduction

Injuries of the wrist have long been recognised but were poorly understood until the early 20th century. With the use of radiography, the descriptions of various fractures and dislocations has encompassed the entire carpus and distal radius.

Treatment of these potentially debilitating injuries has also undergone significant evolution mirroring advances in surgical technique and technology.

Although some of the injuries described are infrequent, their recognition and the subsequent initiation of appropriate treatment significantly reduces morbidity and improves functional outcome. Therefore a basic understanding of the anatomy and biomechanics (which is complex) and the spectrum of injury is recommended for clinicians treating patients with acute wrist injuries.

Anatomy and function

The scaphoid is one of eight carpal bones which lie in two rows (*Figure 15.1*). They are articulated together to form a semicircle, the convexity of which is proximal and articulates with the forearm bones. The scaphoid occupies the most radial position (thumb side) in the proximal row. It is a boat-shaped bone, which articulates directly with the radius proximally and is a critical link in the mechanism of the carpus. It is commonly divided into four distinct parts: the proximal pole, the waist, the distal body and the tuberosity. It is a key bone to both wrist motion and stability.

A complex series of dorsal and volar extrinsic interosseous ligaments exists, the most important being the radioscaphocapitate (volar) and radiotriquetral (dorsal). The intrinsic ligaments run between carpal bones, binding tightly to fix the bones (distal row) or more loosely to allow some intercarpal movement (proximal row): the scapholunate ligament appears to be the primary stabiliser between the scaphoid and lunate and the lunotriquetral ligament between the latter and triquetrum (Berger, 2001).

The blood supply of the scaphoid arises from the radial artery entering the scaphoid at or distal to its waist along the dorsal ridge. This accounts for up to

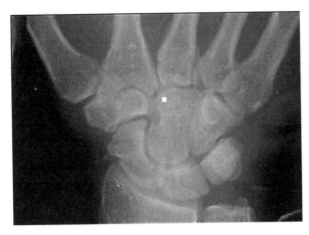

80% of the entire blood supply and as much as 100% of the supply to the proximal pole. Therefore fractures through the waist and proximal third render the more proximal fragment of the scaphoid at risk of avascular necrosis (AVN) or death.

The other bones of the carpus must not be ignored although the scaphoid is the commonest bone to fracture. The carpus serves as a conduit for passage of the wrist and digital motors, providing more mechanical advantage to move the hand on the wrist. When high-energy forces pass through the carpus distal to the radius, soft tissue and bony injuries occur and may cause significant instability patterns.

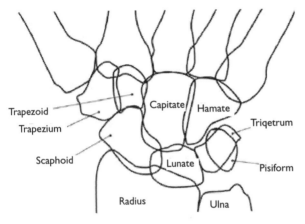

Figure 15.1. Anatomy of the carpus.

Fractures of carpal bones other than the scaphoid usually require referral to orthopaedic teams following stabilisation by plaster of Paris so that instability can be excluded. Important dislocations of carpal bones, mainly the lunate, will be mentioned later in the chapter. The main focus of this section will be the scaphoid.

Mechanisms of injury

Because of its offset proximal and distal articular surfaces, the scaphoid has a natural tendency to palmar-flex with longitudinal loading. Thus, extension of the scaphoid places progressively increasing tension on the palmar cortex of the curved waist of the scaphoid. Excessive extension or ulnar deviation of the wrist, coupled with excessive loading, mechanically predisposes the scaphoid to fracture, especially if the strong ligaments attaching to the scaphoid retain their integrity (Short *et al*, 2002).

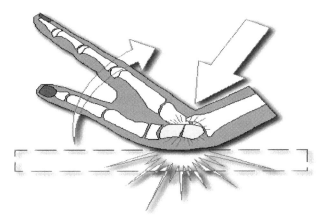

Figure 15.2. Injury to the scaphoid caused by a fall.

Most wrist injuries are incurred by falling on an outstretched hand (*Figure 15.2*). The wrist is usually hyper-extended. Radial or ulnar deviation can determine specific outcome of the injury. Direct trauma may be responsible for hamate hook fractures as can improper swings of sporting equipment. Axial load to the metacarpals can also cause carpal fracture dislocations and rarely, isolated capitate fractures.

Clinical picture and investigations

Most painful wrists are seen in the accident and emergency department where often, inexperienced doctors are assessing the patient. It is important to take a clear and accurate history although this can be difficult. The age and sex of the patient must be taken into account along with the mechanism of injury. Often the painful wrist is examined without comparison to the other side. Many individuals experience pain in the anatomical snuffbox when the superficial radial nerve is compressed. There is much in the literature on how the accurate diagnosis of a scaphoid fracture can be made. These range from the combination of clinical signs, for example, evaluating tenderness in the anatomical snuffbox and over the scaphoid tubercle, pain on longitudinal compression of the thumb and range of thumb movement (Parvizi *et al*, 1998). When these clinical signs were used in combination within the first 24 hours following injury they produced 100% sensitivity and 74% specificity. Failure to diagnose scaphoid fractures that can be well treated acutely, may result in delayed or non-union (with subsequent osteoarthritis) and deformity at a later date. Initial suspicion may be of a distal radial fracture; but if no radial fracture is seen on the preliminary wrist X-rays, then a scaphoid fracture must be suspected.

In the case of other carpal bone fracture, the same principles apply; the carpus may display the obvious deformity of a dislocation. The carpal bones must be examined and palpated individually and a neurovascular assessment performed and documented.

Table 15.1. Differential diagnosis of suspected scaphoid injury

Diagnosis	Physical and radiographic findings
Arthritis of the carpometacarpal or radiocarpal joint	Local tenderness, abnormal radiographs
De Quervain's tenosynovitis	Lateral wrist pain, tenderness over radial styloid, positive Finkelstein's test
Distal radius fracture	Local tenderness and deformity, abnormal plain radiographs
Extensor carpi radialis strain	Local tenderness, swelling, and pain elicited with wrist flexion
First metacarpal fracture	Local tenderness and deformity, abnormal plain radiographs
Flexor carpi radialis strain	Local tenderness, swelling, and pain elicited with wrist extension
Injuries to radioulnar joint	Local tenderness
Scapholunate dissociation	Tenderness over scapholunate ligament, increased gap between scaphoid and lunate on plain films
Scaphoid fracture	Anatomic snuffbox tenderness, pain with scaphoid compression test, tenderness of scaphoid tubercle

Due to the complex anatomy of the scaphoid at least four views on plain X-ray are required to show the bone adequately (scaphoid views). Despite four views these can still be difficult to interpret and consequently some fractures are missed. If no fracture is seen but highly suspected, the patient is commonly placed in a scaphoid cast and asked to return one week to 10 days later for a follow-up X-ray. The fracture is often diagnosed at this juncture when the X-rays are more likely to show a fracture line, but inevitably a proportion are still not evident – missed or true negatives.

If the diagnosis cannot be established by clinical and simple radiographic means, bone scans have been recommended in the literature and preferred over computed tomography (CT) or magnetic resonance imaging (MRI) for expense reasons. MRI allows an early definitive diagnosis to be made and should be regarded as the gold standard investigation. MRI also has the advantage of being the best investigation to determine avascular necrosis, in the longer term, while CT has an established role in detecting non-unions. See *Table 15.1* for the differential diagnosis of suspected scaphoid injury.

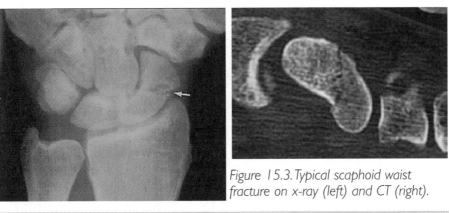

Figure 15.3. Typical scaphoid waist fracture on x-ray (left) and CT (right).

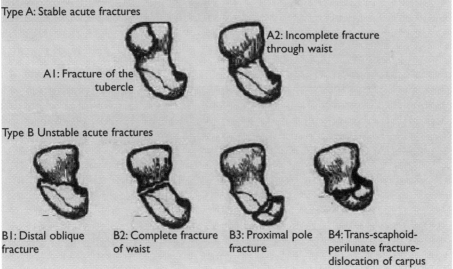

Type A: Stable acute fractures

A1: Fracture of the tubercle

A2: Incomplete fracture through waist

Type B Unstable acute fractures

B1: Distal oblique fracture

B2: Complete fracture of waist

B3: Proximal pole fracture

B4: Trans-scaphoid-perilunate fracture-dislocation of carpus

Figure 15.4. Herbert classification of scaphoid fractures.

Common fractures and dislocations

Approximately 50% of fractures of the scaphoid occur across the waist (*Figure 15.3*); about 38% of fractures occur in the proximal half and 12% in the distal half.

Classification

Two methods of classifying scaphoid fractures are recognised. Russe in 1960 described the fractures in three types, based on the relationship of the fracture line to the long axis of the scaphoid: transverse, vertical oblique and horizontal

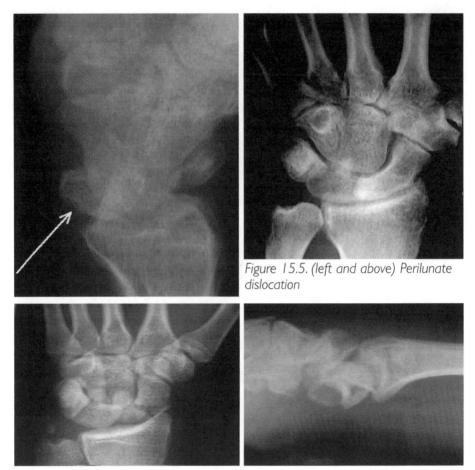

Figure 15.5. (left and above) Perilunate dislocation

Figure 15.6. Trans-scapho perilunate dislocation.

oblique. Herbert and Fisher in 1984 classified scaphoid fractures more broadly (*Figure 15.4*) as unstable or stable; stable fractures include crack fractures and tuberosity fractures; unstable fractures include distal third, proximal pole and displaced waist fractures, as well as fractures associated with carpal dislocation and comminuted fractures.

It should be noted that marked displacement of a fractured scaphoid can be associated with carpal dislocation.

Dislocations of the carpus fall into two main groups. In the first, the metacarpals, the distal row of the carpus and part of the proximal row dislocate dorsally; the prefix 'peri' is used to describe undisplaced structures in the proximal row (commonly the lunate), eg. perilunate dislocation of the carpus (*Figure 15.5*), periscapholunate dislocation and trans-scaphoid perilunate dislocation of the carpus (*Figure 15.6*). The latter involves a fracture of the scaphoid in addition to a perilunar dislocation. In the second group, the distal

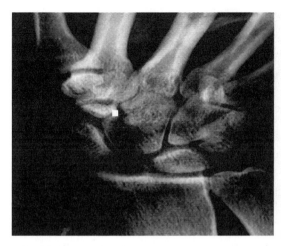

Figure 15.7. Scapholunate
dissociation ('Terry Thomas' sign).

row re-aligns with the radius and part of the proximal row is extruded; these tend to be pure dislocations of a carpal bone, eg. scaphoid, lunate (the commonest), lunate and scaphoid or lunate and part of the scaphoid.

Finally scapholunate dissociation (*Figure 15.7*) needs to be mentioned. This occurs when attachments of the lunate and the scaphoid have been completely lost by either fracture of the scaphoid or complete rupture of the scapholunate interosseous ligaments. Subtle changes on the X-ray are seen including widening of the intercarpal space with or without a fracture. Pain may be global acutely and sub-acute examination may yield more information in terms of point tenderness and ballottment or shift of the bones involved (Kirk-Watson test). This is an important diagnosis to make as the long-term sequelae of this injury result in pain, deformity, loss of normal function and ultimately osteoarthritis.

Management

Initial

If there is any doubt over the injury in this area, orthopaedic opinion should be sought. Interpretation of X-rays can be difficult, especially in dislocations. If dislocation is seen, then mandatory referral is recommended.

For undisplaced scaphoid fractures, no reduction is required. Importance is placed on the application of an appropriate plaster cast – a below elbow cast with a thumb spica essentially; however the wrist should be fully pronated, radially deviated, moderately dorsiflexed and the thumb in mid-abduction. Moreover interphalangeal movement of the thumb should not be restricted. The patient should be reviewed in an orthopaedic clinic in a week.

Dislocations generally require reduction under general anaesthesia. They frequently also require fixation either percutaneously or internally so should be

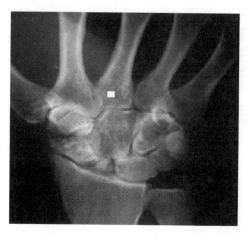

Figure 15.8. Scaphoid non-union.

referred urgently, particularly if there is neurological compromise. Temporary stabilisation in a volar plaster of Paris slab is adequate. A sling for elevation for reduction of swelling is helpful.

Definitive

Undisplaced scaphoid fractures are casted for six weeks. X-ray after cast removal demonstrating union is sought. Clinical assessment is then performed. If adverse symptomology persists, however, it is not uncommon practice to allow further time in a cast for union to occur; this may be up to four further weeks. However prolonged time in a cast has significant disadvantages, particularly for athletes and young employed adults, and thus signs of delayed union or non-union (*Figure 15.8*) at 8–10 weeks may signal the need for operative intervention. Displaced fracture union rates are less and lower thresholds for operative intervention predominate.

Operative options are open reduction and internal fixation with or without bone grafting, commonly with an intra-osseous screw (*Figure 15.9*), or closed manipulation and percutaneous fixation (*Figure 15.10*). Both techniques have good success and choice is surgeon dependent (Inoue and Shionoya, 1997; Haddad and Goddard, 1998).

Longer-term follow up of this group of patients is paramount as late avascular necrosis is a well recognised late complication (particularly in waist and proximal pole fractures), which may be diagnosed by MRI and will require further operative intervention.

Conclusion

The anatomy and biomechanics of the carpus represent a subject of immense complexity. A thorough understanding is unnecessary provided some important

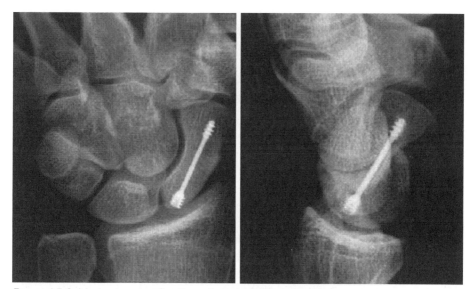

Figure 15.9. Herbert screw fixation of a scaphoid waist fracture.

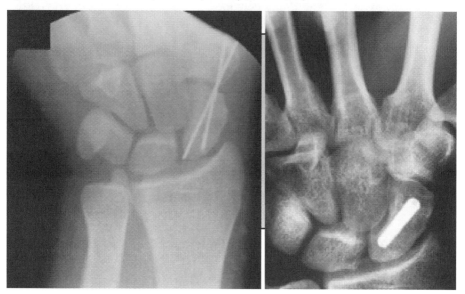

Figure 15.10. Percutaneous fixation of a scaphoid waist fracture.

principles are considered (see *Key points*). It also should be borne in mind that carpal injuries usually follow distinct patterns, linked to the mechanism of injury. Radiographic evidence of injury can be subtle and some injuries do not manifest immediately on X-ray. If there is any doubt about the diagnosis, expert orthopaedic opinion should be sought as the long-term morbidity of missing such injuries can be devastating.

Key points

- The scaphoid is a boat-shaped bone, which articulates directly with the radius proximally and is a critical link in the mechanism of the carpus.
- The blood supply of the scaphoid arises from the radial artery entering the scaphoid at or distal to its waist along the dorsal ridge. This accounts for up to 80% of the entire blood supply. Therefore fractures through the waist and proximal third render the more proximal fragment of the scaphoid at risk of avascular necrosis.
- The carpus serves as a conduit for passage of the wrist and digital motors, providing more mechanical advantage to move the hand on the wrist.
- Most wrist injuries are incurred by falling on an outstretched hand. The wrist is usually hyperextended. Radial or ulnar deviation can determine specific outcome of the injury.
- Accurate diagnosis of a scaphoid fracture can be made by evaluating tenderness in the anatomical snuffbox and over the scaphoid tubercle, pain on longitudinal compression of the thumb and range of thumb movement.
- If no fracture is seen but highly suspected, the patient is placed in a scaphoid cast and asked to return one week to 10 days later for a follow-up X-ray. The fracture is often diagnosed at this juncture when the X-rays are more likely to show a fracture line.
- MRI allows an early definitive diagnosis to be made and should be regarded as the gold standard investigation.
- It should be noted that marked displacement of a fractured scaphoid can be associated with carpal dislocation.
- For undisplaced scaphoid fractures, no reduction is required. Importance is placed on the application of an appropriate plaster cast – a below elbow cast with a thumb spica essentially; however the wrist should be fully pronated, radially deviated, moderately dorsiflexed and the thumb in mid-abduction.

References

Berger RA (2001) The anatomy of the scaphoid. *Hand Clin* **17**: 525–32

Haddad FS,.Goddard NJ (1998) Acute percutaneous scaphoid fixation. A pilot study. *J Bone Joint Surg (Br)* **80**: 95–9

Herbert TJ, Fisher WE (1984) Management of scaphoid injury using a new bone screw. *J Bone Joint Surg Br* **66(1)**: 114–23

Inoue G, Shionoya K (1997) Herbert screw fixation by limited access for acute fractures of the scaphoid. *J Bone Joint Surg (Br)* **79**: 418–21

Parvizi J, Wayman J, Kelly P, Moran CG (1998) Combining the clinical signs improves diagnosis of scaphoid fractures. A prospective study with follow-up. *J Hand Surg (Br)* **23**: 324–7

Russe O (1960) Fractures of the carpal navicular. Diagnosis, non-operative treatment and operative treatment. *J Bone Joint Surg Am* **42-A**: 759–68

Short WH, Werner FW, Green JK, Masaoka S (2002) Biomechanical evaluation of ligamentous stabilizers of the scaphoid and lunate. *J Hand Surg (Am)* **27**: 991–1002

CHAPTER 16

Metacarpal and phalangeal injuries

Nicholas Wardle and Fares Haddad

Introduction

Injuries to the hand are common with phalangeal and metacarpal fractures accounting for 10% of all fractures. The resulting morbidity from delayed treatment to hand injuries is particularly high in the dominant hand. A brief overview of the salient conditions is presented here.

Anatomy

The small joints of the hand are hinged joints. The metacarpophalangeal (MCP) joints have a 'cam' configuration, whereas the proximal interphalangeal (PIP) and distal interphalangeal (DIP) joints have a spherical shape. Stability depends not only on the articular contour but on the collateral ligaments and volar plate. The volar plate is a thick fibrocartilaginous portion of the volar capsule that connects the neck of the bone proximal to the joint to the base of the bone distal to the joint. The volar plate has strong lateral attachments but a weak distal attachment.

Owing to the eccentricity of the metacarpal head the collateral ligaments are more taught in flexion than in extension, and therefore the MCP joint needs to be immobilised in flexion.

Small joint injuries

A partial or complete tear of the collateral ligaments, volar plate, or extensor tendon results in subluxation or dislocation of the finger joint. Intra-articular fractures, including avulsion fractures and fracture dislocations, may be associated with these injuries.

Evaluation of swelling, tenderness or bruising of a finger should raise concerns that a joint injury has occurred. Ligamentous injury often causes instability which can be assessed by stress testing – ensure the comparative non-injured opposite side is tested where possible to help distinguish from ligament laxity.

Limited motion may arise from joint subluxation or displaced articular fractures, it is therefore imperative that good quality radiographs are obtained and these should include anteroposterior (AP), direct lateral and possibly an oblique view.

Common DIP joint injuries

Mallet finger

Mallet finger results from sudden forced flexion to the DIP causing extensor tendon rupture from the distal phalanx (± bony fragment). With an appropriate history such as catching the finger in clothing and the resulting clinical picture of pain, swelling and tenderness coupled with an inability to actively extend the joint the diagnosis should be relatively straightforward. Radiographs are often unhelpful but may show an avulsed fragment of bone. Large fracture fragments (>30%) of the articular surface are at risk of volar subluxation of the distal phalanx. Initial management is aimed at determining the severity of any avulsed bony fragment with radiographic assessment, this then dictates either simple treatment with splinting/casting for mallet fingers with <30% fracture fragments or displaced less than 2mm, or need for surgical intervention – for >30% fragment size, >2mm displacement or associated with volar subluxation of the distal phalanx

Dorsal DIP joint dislocation

Dorsal DIP joint dislocation hyperextension to the tip of the finger may disrupt the volar plate and collateral ligaments. The injury is frequently associated with volar laceration, owing to the adherence of the volar skin to the underlying bone. Initial management is to attempt closed reduction under a digital block (ensure that no adrenaline is in the local anaesthetic used for this purpose) and, if successful, splint the joint with either neighbour strapping or a rigid splint for between 2–4 weeks. Dislocations associated with significant volar skin lacerations with suspicion of compromise to the joint, or irreducible dislocations require surgical intervention with open reduction with or without repair to the collateral ligaments or volar plate with subsequent splintage then hand therapy to promote range of motion.

Common PIP joint injuries

Collateral ligament sprain

Either abduction or adduction forces applied to an extended finger can cause tearing of the collateral ligaments. The radial collateral ligament is injured more frequently than the ulnar. Tenderness over the site of injury is seen and stress testing should be performed in 20° of flexion; lack of firm end-point is diagnostic of a complete tear. Radiographs can demonstrate small chip fractures, and record the degree of angulation under stress testing. Partial and most complete tears can be treated with static splinting (1–2 weeks) and then neighbour strapping (further 3 weeks). Surgical intervention is indicated when radiographic evidence of soft tissue interposition is noted, when there is a displaced condylar fracture of middle phalanx, or when closed treatment fails.

Volar plate injury
A hyperextension force to the PIP may cause the volar plate to tear from the middle phalanx (± bony fragment). Closed management is indicated in stable injuries with dorsal splinting (in 20° of flexion) for 1 week.

Dorsal PIP dislocation
Dorsal PIP dislocation is one of the most frequently seen articular injuries to the hand. Hyperextension at the PIP joint results in dislocation of the middle phalanx dorsally. Closed treatment with reduction and neighbour strapping for 3–6 weeks is usual, although the presence of a volar fragment >15% of articular surface may require operative intervention.

Common MCP joint injuries

Thumb MCP ulnar collateral ligament injury
This injury is also known as 'gamekeeper's thumb' or 'ski-pole thumb'. Competency of the ulnar collateral ligament is essential for effective lateral key pinch. Stress testing should be performed comparing with the un-injured thumb, and stress radiographs indicating >35° of opening suggest a complete tear. Closed treatment is indicated in partial tears with good end-points and not opening more than 35°. Cast immobilisation for 4–6 weeks is used. Surgical treatment is for the unstable, complete tear or those with a displaced fracture fragment.

Metacarpal fractures

Metacarpal fractures account for a third of all fractures in the hand.

Classification

Described by location; including metacarpal head, neck, shaft and base. Typically subclassified into non-displaced or displaced, closed or open, and associated with angulation, rotation or shortening deformity.

Management

Physical examination
Remove all jewellery. Check for:

- obvious deformity
- bruising/swelling
- pain and tenderness to palpation
- restricted range of motion
- malrotation/angulation of digits
- vascular/nerve involvement.

Radiographic evaluation
AP and lateral views of the metacarpal bones are used to define fracture alignment. A tangential (Brewertons) view is useful for evaluating metacarpal head fractures.

Metacarpal head fractures
Non-displaced head fractures can be treated with either neighbour strapping or cast protection. Displaced oblique fractures require Open reduction and internal fixation (ORIF) with either Kirschner wires or small screws. There is a possibility that avascular necrosis may still occur in the metacarpal head even after a non-displaced transverse fracture.

Metacarpal neck fractures
Also known as 'boxers' fractures. As a result of a direct blow on the metacarpal head (usually of the ring or little finger) the metacarpal neck may fracture with associated angulation. If the angulation is less than 15° the fracture can be treated conservatively (neighbour strapping/ulnar gutter cast). For angulation between 15°–40° the fracture requires reduction with subsequent ulnar gutter splintage. Above 40° of angulation closed reduction and percutaneous wiring is indicated. Residual angulation of more than 15° is unacceptable in the index and long fingers, as there is a lack of compensatory carpometacarpal motion for these fingers. However a total of 40° dorsal angulation can be accepted in the little finger.

Metacarpal shaft fractures
Transverse shaft fractures often result from a direct blow to the hand, these fractures can be treated conservatively with reduction and cast application. Spiral and long oblique fractures of the shaft are unstable with shortening and rotation. ORIF is indicated for shaft fractures that have malrotation, dorsal angulation >10° for index and middle fingers, dorsal angulation >20° for ring

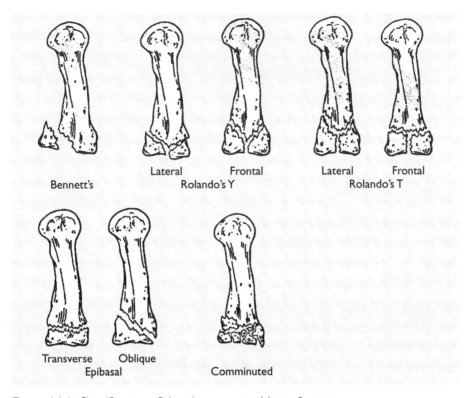

Bennett's

Lateral   Frontal
Rolando's Y

Lateral   Frontal
Rolando's T

Transverse   Oblique
Epibasal

Comminuted

Figure 16.1. Classification of thumb metacarpal base fractures.

and little fingers and any shortening greater than 3mm. In multiple metacarpal shaft fractures it is recommended that internal fixation is performed.

Metacarpal base fractures

Stable base fractures can be treated in just a cast, however displaced fractures require closed reduction and percutaneous fixation.

Thumb metacarpal base fractures

Fractures in this region can affect lateral key pinch and opposition of the thumb to other digits. This group of fractures are classified separately into (*Figure 16. 1*)

* Bennett's fracture-dislocation
* Rolando's Y or T condylar fracture
* epibasal fracture
* comminuted fracture.

There is notable swelling and pain at the base of the thumb, commonly associated with bruising in the thenar region.

Treatment depends upon whether the fracture is displaced or not. Non-displaced fractures that are in good alignment can be treated with a cast for 4 weeks. Displaced fractures require either percutaneous wiring or ORIF, as only 1–3mm of carpometacarpal incongruity can be accepted.

Phalangeal fractures

In combination phalangeal and metacarpal fractures account for nearly 10% of all fractures.

Classification

Extra-articular phalangeal fractures are classified the same as metacarpal fractures, but include a tuft fracture for the distal phalanx.

Examination

Remove all jewellery. Radiographic evaluation should be prompted by swelling, pain, limited motion and deformity. Up to 30% of phalangeal fractures are open injuries. Obtain AP and lateral radiographs (fingers need to be splayed and in varying degrees of flexion to obtain good lateral views).

Management

As with all fractures accurate reduction is vital to allow normal function. Fingers need to be mobilised as soon as fracture stability allows to prevent debilitating stiffness; those fingers not involved in the injury should be mobilised as soon as possible for the same reason. The PIP joint is the most important joint for motion and function of the digit.

Stable fractures
If well aligned stable fractures can be treated with neighbour strapping, splint or cast.

Displaced fractures
If reduction is possible and stability can be maintained then treatment with a cast or splint is advocated. However it may be necessary to use percutaneous wiring to prevent the fracture from displacing again.

Unstable fractures
If, despite attempted closed reduction, position and stability cannot be maintained then ORIF is indicated. Options include K-wires, interfragmentary

screws or plate and screw fixation. If there is segmental bone loss then external fixation may be required.

Conclusion

It is imperative that injuries to the hand and fingers are diagnosed promptly and correctly enabling the correct treatment to be instigated. If an injury is missed the resulting impact on the function of the hand can be devastating, particularly if the injury occurred in the dominant hand.

Careful evaluation of the injured region and radiographs are required as often the diagnosis is not straightforward – especially in respect to ligamentous injuries.

Key points

- Phalangeal and metacarpal fractures account for 10% of all fractures.
- Ligamentous injuries are relatively easy to overlook in the acutely injured hand.
- Careful radiograph evaluation is required when dealing with intra-articular injuries.
- Early mobilisation is required to allow any chance of return to normal functioning of an injured digit.
- Rotational malalignment is a common problem with hand fractures and must not be overlooked.

Further reading

Brinker MR, Miller MD (1999) *Fundamentals of Orthopaedics*. WB Saunders, Philadelphia

Schenck RR (1994) The dynamic traction method combining movement and. traction for intra-articular fractures of the phalanges. *Hand Clin* **10(2)**: 187–98

CHAPTER 17

Hand injuries and infections

Max Horwitz and Elliot Sorene

Anatomy and function

The hand may be looked upon as a complex soft tissue envelope with a bony skeleton to support intricate function. Function follows the restitution of form in the hand.

It is worth spending some time familiarising oneself with the anatomy of the hand. The hand is made up of 27 bones. The carpus is separated from the distal radius and ulna by an ellipsoid joint. The proximal row of the carpus includes the scaphoid, lunate, triquetral and a piso-triquetral articulation. The distal includes the trapezium, trapezoid, capitate and hamate. All of the carpal bones except the pisiform are gliding joints. The carpometarcarpal (CMC) joint of the thumb is a highly mobile saddle joint. The other CMC joints are ellipsoid. The interphalangeal joints are hinges. Each finger is made up of three phalanges while the thumb only has two.

The joints are generally supported by strong collateral ligaments as well as dorsal and volar ligaments (which in certain places are condensed to volar plates). These structures prevent excessive hyper-extension and radial/ulna deviation.

The hand contains both intrinsic and extrinsic muscles. The intrinsic muscles originate and insert along the metacarpals. The four dorsal interossei abduct the fingers and assist with metacarpophalangeal joint (MCPJ) flexion. The three palmar interossei adduct the fingers and aid MCPJ flexion as well as interphalangeal joint extension. They are all supplied by the deep branch of the ulnar nerve.

There are four lumbrical muscles which arise from the side of the flexor digitorum profundus (FDP) tendon. They terminate on the lateral slips of the extensor tendons. The lumbricals flex the MCP joints and extend the interphalangeal joints. The radial two lumbricals are supplied by the median nerve and the ulna two by the ulna nerve.

Each finger has two flexor tendons. The FDP inserts on the base of the distal phalanx and passes through the flexor digitorum superficialis (FDS) which inserts on the middle phalanx. They run through a sheath and five annular pulleys (between joints) as well as three cruciate pulleys at the joints (*Figure 17.1*) (Boyer *et al*, 2002). The tendons were divided into zones by Kleinert and Verdan in 1983. The prognosis for repair is different in each zone

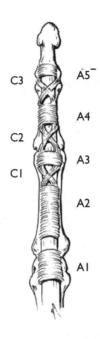

C3
C2
C1

Á5⁻
A4
A3
A2
A1

Figure 17.1. (left) Pulley system of the flexor tendons; A: annular; C: cruciate.

Figure 17.2. (right) Flexor tendon zones:
Zone I: Distal to the DIPJ.
Zone II: Under the A2 pulley.
Zone III: Proximal to the A2 pulley in the palm.
Zone IV: Under the flexor retinaculum.
Zone V: In the forearm.

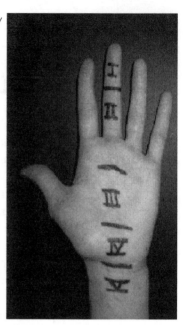

(*Figure 17.2*) (Hayton, 2002). The thumb has a solitary flexor tendon but also has other structures to enable opposition, adduction and abduction.

There are six extensor compartments at the wrist. These tendons ensure wrist, thumb and finger extension and, in the case of the thumb, abduction. The tendons divide into three slips over the MCP joints. The middle slip connects to the proximal phalanx via the sagittal bands. This ensures proximal phalangeal extension. The tendon then goes on to attach to the middle phalanx and extends it in turn. The two lateral slips unite and insert onto the base of the distal phalanx to extend it. (*Figure 17.3*) (Tubiana and Valentin, 1964; Bendre *et al*, 2005) The extensor tendons are also divided into zones.

The hand is supplied by the radial and ulna arteries which form the deep and superficial palmar arches respectively. Each finger has radial and ulna digital arteries.

The median nerve supplies the sensation to the volar aspect of the radial three and a half fingers as well as the centre of the palm. The ulna nerve supplies the ulna volar of one and a half fingers. The superficial branch of the radial nerve supplies the dorsum of the hand.

The fingertip and nail have specialised anatomy. The skin of the pulp must be robust yet highly sensate. The pulp consists of fibro-fatty tissue. The nail plate rests on a nail bed and originates from the germinal matrix. The surrounding skin on the dorsum of the nail is known as the paronychium. It is essential to refer to the correct portions of the fingertip when describing any injuries.

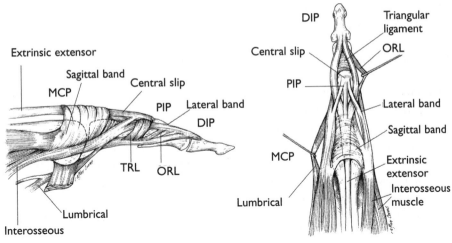

Figure 17.3. Extensor anatomy.
DIP: distal interphalangeal joint; MCP: metacarpophalangeal joint; PIP: proximal interphalangeal joint; TRL: transverse retinacular ligament; ORL: oblique retinacular ligament.

Mechanism of injury and clinical findings

It is essential to ascertain the exact time the injury occurred, how it occurred and which object if any caused the damage. An injury with a clean blade is very different to an injury with a soil-covered farm tool or a crushing injury. The position of the hand at the time of injury is also important. If a flexor tendon is cut in flexion, the distal portion will retract aonce the hand is opened. If the hand was cut in extension the distal portion tends to stay put.

A history of any life-threatening injuries must be taken and acted upon according to Advanced Trauma Life Support (ATLS) protocols. Hand dominance, occupation, hobbies and medical history must be noted. Tetanus status must be checked and updated if necessary. A booster is usually adequate unless there is a high risk of tetanus, in which case a vaccine is given. A history of substance abuse and self-harm are also vital in the long-term management of hand injuries.

A methodical examination must take place. It is often helpful to alleviate pain with a local block but nervous status must be documented prior to this. The skin, tendons, ligaments, joints and bones must all be systematically evaluated. It is best to describe the fingers as middle, index, ring and little rather then one, two, three and four. Digital photographs with consent are very useful.

Skin wounds

Skin loss and devitalised tissue must be noted. After local wound toilet a limited exploration should take place. Hand wounds often look superficial but the underlying structures are equally superficial. Glass is renowned for causing small wounds but there may be large underlying tissue damage, especially with high energy injuries.

Vascular injury

Capillary refill is a very good indication of vascular perfusion. A grey mottled finger with a delayed refill (>2 seconds) cannot be ignored. Fortunately the bilateral supply of blood to most digits prevents ischaemia. Allen's test is employed to assess the arterial supply to the hand. The test is performed by compressing the radial and ulna arteries at the wrist with digital pressure. The patient is then asked to make a fist several times. The hand will blanch. On release of one of the arteries the hand and fingers will go pink indicating good flow in the released vessel and good collateral flow into the occluded vessel. The test is considered positive if the hand fails to reperfuse. Heavy arterial bleeding usually stops with pressure and elevation. There is no place for the haphazard placement of artery clips in the emergency department. These wounds should be properly explored if the bleeding does not stop.

Nerve injury

Patients usually report cutting themselves with a knife or other sharp object. The sensory and motor function of all nerves must be documented prior to local anaesthetic block. Two point discrimination is a useful test for assessing sensory deficit. A paperclip can be separated to 5mm and the digit tested for discrimination on the finger pulp; 15mm is recommended for the dorsum of the hand. An absence of sweating is another indicator of a nerve injury. In polytrauma it is always important to examine the neck and the rest of the upper limb.

Flexor tendon injury

The majority of flexor tendon injuries are due to sharp objects lacerating the tendon. Occasionally the FDP insertion can be avulsed at its insertion. This is known as a 'rugby jersey' injury. Examination of the hand at rest is the first step. A loss of the normal finger cascade is a tell tale sign (*Figure 17.4*). This cascade can be demonstrated in unconscious patients due to the tenodesis effect, where passive extension of the flexed wrist should result in finger flexion. Complete tendon injuries are usually apparent while incomplete injuries can pose a diagnostic challenge. Pain in a finger is a very useful guide. A brief exploration of the wound after toilet is also helpful.

The FDP is tested by actively flexing the distal interphalangeal joint (DIPJ) while the examiner holds the proximal interphalangeal joint (PIPJ) in a fixed position. The FDS of the middle, ring and little finger is tested by placing the

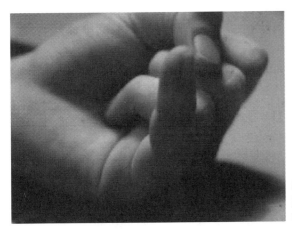

Figure 17. 4. Loss of the normal finger cascade following flexor tendon injury to the little finger.

hand flat on the table and pressing the non-affected fingers flat while allowing the affected finger to flex at the MCPJ. The index finger may be tested in this manner but it is best to test it by pinching it to the thumb with an extended DIPJ. If the FDS is absent then the FDP will compensate by flexing the DIPJ and creating a pinch grip.

Extensor tendon injury

The most common type of injury is a mallet finger. These were classified by Doyle (1999) and are usually caused by hyper-extension at the DIPJ but can be secondary to an open laceration of the extensor tendon or a fracture at the insertion. The finger must be checked for an inability to extend – an extensor lag. The central slip can be tested by performing Elson's test (Elson, 1986): the PIPJ is held in flexion and the patient is asked to extend the DIPJ. Inability to extend may be a sign of a central slip injury.

Ligament and joint injury

Dislocated interphalangeal joints are a common injury. They occur during forceful hyperextension or wrenching in a radial or ulna direction. After acute reduction it is very important to assess the stability of the joint as well as tendon function. Plain radiographs are essential. The ulna aspect of the thumb has a very important ulna collateral ligament. This is important for pinch grip. Forced abduction can tear this ligament. It should be tested by abducting the thumb at the MCPJ level at both 30° of flexion and extension. It is important to compare it to the other side. A local anaesthetic block is often very useful to aid examination. High energy injuries can also disrupt the intercarpal ligaments. These injuries can result in long-term instability and occasionally very serious dislocation such as per-lunate dislocation.

Bony injury

A third of all skeletal fractures occur in the hand. The hand is used reflexively for protection and often takes the brunt of an injury. All 27 bones of the hand should be palpated. A clinical assessment of rotation and alignment should be performed. On finger flexion all of the fingernails should point to the scaphoid. There should be no crossing over of fingers. A patient will usually be able to localise pain to a specific bone. The majority of hand fractures are treated conservatively. Splintage and early mobilisation is a good treatment method for the majority of stable fractures. Intra-articular and unstable fractures may need surgery.

Fingertip and nail bed injuries

Fingertips are often caught in doors or crushed by other means. It is important to assess whether the nail has come loose from the proximal nail fold and whether or not there is a nail bed injury. A radiograph is essential to exclude a tuft fracture. It is also important to check for a mallet injury.

Clinical picture and investigations

All of the above must be added together to try and create a clear picture regarding the severity of the injury and the resultant lack of function. Further management depends on this decision. The majority of hand injuries (which make up at least a fifth of accident and emergency attendances) can be treated in casualty and discharged home.

Plain radiographs are usually adequate. These include anteroposterior (AP) and lateral views. Scaphoid views must be requested if there is a suspicion of a scaphoid fracture. True lateral views are very important in assessing joint congruity especially in PIPJ and DIPJ injuries. It is often necessary to get an oblique view to properly assess the 4th and 5th metacarpals. Radiographs should also be considered when there are penetrating or glass injuries.

Specific problems

Infection

Hand infections can be devastating and must be taken seriously. It is not within the scope of this book to discuss them in depth. However a few basic principles if adhered to will guide the clinician in the initial consultation. If infection is suspected swabs of any pus should be sent for microbiological assessment and broad spectrum intravenous antibiotics should be started through a cannula

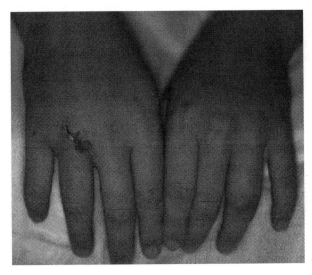

Figure 17.5. The 'fight bite'.

placed in the contralateral limb. There is often severe swelling and redness with pain on passive movement.

A special mention must be made regarding the 'fight bite' (*Figure 17.5*) (Chuinard and Ambrosia, 1977). This refers to lacerations usually over the MCPJ. These injuries are sustained when a hand is punched into a mouth and a sharp tooth penetrates the skin often all the way into the joint. Infection can be sudden and severe. The patient should be X-rayed and must be referred for debridement, joint lavage and intravenous antibiotics.

Fractures

If, after reduction, splintage and check radiograph, there is significant shortening, angulation and/or malrotation with intra-articular incongruity the patient should be referred for possible surgical intervention.(*Figure 17.6*). It is essential to include the joint above and below the fracture in radiographs.

It is not always possible to tell whether there is an acute fracture of the scaphoid bone. If in doubt the hand should be immobilised in plaster and the patient should have repeat radiographs two weeks later.

High pressure injection injury

High pressure injection equipment can penetrate the skin and cause devastating underlying tissue damage (*Figure 17.7*). The wounds are often very small but a history and extreme pain should arouse suspicion. The fingers are typically very swollen with diminished sensation. It is useful to find out what was injected and refer on an urgent basis for surgical debridement.

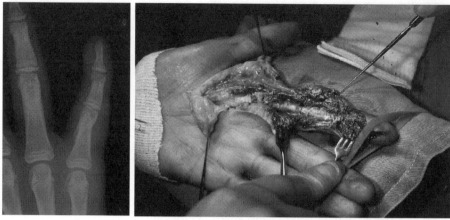

Figure 17.6. (left) A displaced intra-articular fracture of the proximal phalanx of the little finger. Figure 17.7. (right) High pressure injection injury causing widespread tissue damage.

Ring avulsion

The ring is caught, commonly on a fence. It is pulled distally, degloving bony tissues from the skeleton of the finger. This can lead to vascular compromise and must be urgently referred after X-ray (*Figure 17.8*).

Burns

Superficial burns (painful, sensate with capillary refill less than 2 seconds) can be treated with analgesia and early mobilisation. All other burns should be referred to the hand surgery or burn team. Chemical burns must be treated with extensive irrigation after consultation with a local poisons centre.

Amputation

Amputated digits can survive for 12 hours and this can be extended to 24 hours if kept cold. Amputated digits should be kept in saline and placed in double sealed plastic bags. The bag should be kept in iced water not directly on ice. The amputated part should be X-rayed.

Compartment syndrome

This occurs when the pressure within a closed fascial compartment exceeds the capillary perfusion pressure. It may be secondary to severe fractures, burns, prolonged compression and vascular injury. The most important signs and symptoms of compartment syndrome are pain on passive stretching of the digits

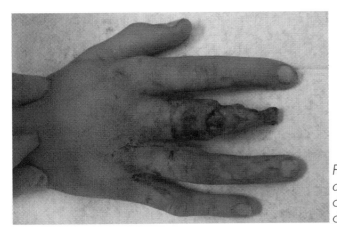

Figure 17.8: A ring avulsion injury with degloving of tissues distal to the ring.

and pain out of proportion to the injury despite analgesia. If this diagnosis is being considered then urgent referral to the surgical team must be made.

Accident and emergency management

The majority of open wounds can be sutured in the emergency department. A senior or orthopaedic opinion should be sought immediately if there is:

- Vascular compromise or suspicion of imminent vascular compromise.
- Amputation or ring avulsion.
- Uncontrolled source of bleeding which is potentially compromising, eg. from the ulna or radial artery.
- Neurological damage.
- Digit or limb-threatening infection (eg. flexor tenosynovitis, necrotising fasciitis) or sepsis.
- Compartment syndrome.
- High pressure injection injury.

The following guidelines should be adhered to for all wounds:

- Tetanus, prophylaxis, with or without immunoglobulin.
- Antibiotic cover for open fractures. (Oral for tuft fractures associated with nail bed injuries, intravenous for all other open fractures.)
- Wash all wounds, whether or not they are going to be explored.
- Do not explore a wound if it definitely needs to go to theatre anyway or if you are not confident of what you are doing.
- Explore if it will change management, such as: a small piece of glass in the wound on X-ray, no other neurovascular or tenderness injury, and you are confident of removing foreign bodies while skin cover is not compromised.

Dressings should be non-adhesive and should not immobilise uninjured joints. Patients should be sent home with advice on elevation while finger, shoulder and elbow range of motion exercises should be encouraged. Follow up at an appropriate clinic must be arranged to remove sutures as well as to assess mobility. Stiffness can occur very quickly and early mobilisation is essential.

The majority of hand fractures can be treated by appropriate splintage or manipulation under local anaesthetic blockade in the emergency department. It is imperative that an X-ray is taken after manipulation or splintage. Elevation advice must be provided and a follow up in a fracture clinic must be booked. Radiograph interpretation can be difficult and if in doubt senior consultation should take place. Specific unstable fractures (as previously mentioned) should be directly referred to the hand surgery team.

Further management

Serious wounds are explored and debrided in the operating theatre. It may be necessary to skin graft or perform local flaps to cover skin defects. The majority of fingertip injuries are suitable for healing by secondary intention after the nail bed has been repaired.

Infections with collections of pus such as flexor sheath or deep space infections require thorough surgical drainage and debridement and often require more than one visit to the operating theatre. This is especially true for the 'fight bite' injury.

If tendon injury is significant (>50–60%) then repair and splintage takes place. Patients can expect to be splinted for six weeks and often undergo lengthy periods of rehabilitation. Nerves are repaired under magnification.

Unstable joint injuries are either treated with splintage alone or a combination of anatomical repair with protective wire fixation. Open fractures are debrided and stabilised in theatre. Specific fracture types can be treated with internal fixation but patient compliance with hand therapy and splintage after surgery is essential.

Key points

- Mechanism of injury is important to plan treatment.
- Tendon injuries often occur at the same time as nerve and vascular injuries.
- Plain radiographs are mandatory for all significant soft tissue injuries.
- Elevation and mobilisation of injured joints is essential.
- Early recognition of hand infections can prevent much morbidity and even mortality.

References:

Bendre AA, Hartigan BJ, Kalainov DMJ (2005) Mallet finger. *Am Acad Orthop Surg* **13**: 336–44

Boyer MI, Strickland JW, Engles DR, Sachar K, Leversedge FJ (2002) Flexor tendon repair and rehabilitation: State of the art in 2002. *J Bone Joint Surg Am* **84**: 1684–706

Chuinard R, Ambrosia D (1977) Human bite infections of the hand. *J Bone Joint Surg Am* **59(3)**: 416–8

Doyle RD (1999) Extensor tendons: Acute injuries. In Green DP, Hotchkiss RT, Pederson WC. (eds) *Green's Operative Hand Surgery*. 4th Edn. Churchill Livingstone, Philadelphia

Elson RA (1986) Rupture of the central slip of the extensor hood of the finger. A test for early diagnosis. *J Bone Joint Surg* **68-B(2)**: 229–31

Hayton M (2002) Mini-symposium: The frauamatised hand. Assessment of hand injuries. *Curr Orthop* **16**: 246–54

Kleinert HE, Verdan C (1983) Report of the committee on tendon injuries. *J Hand Surg* **8(5)**: 794–8

Tubiana R, Valentin P (1964) The anatomy of the extensor apparatus of the fingers. *Surg Clin North Am* **44**: 897–906

CHAPTER 18

Fracture of the proximal femur

Claire Young and Fares Haddad

Introduction

There are approximately 40 000 admissions a year across the UK of patients with fractured proximal femora (Bottle and Alylin, 2006). The incidence of femoral neck fracture increases with age and is more common in females. Osteoporosis (and associated conditions) is a major risk factor and any condition which predisposes the patient to frequent falls plays a considerable role. Such is the socio-economic cost, morbidity and mortality of proximal femoral fractures that there are now guidelines in place for the treatment of osteoporosis (British Orthopaedic Association, 2003; NICE, 2005) and thus prevention of such injuries. It is important to bear in mind that fractured neck of femur and its sequelae represent a significant proportion of hospital deaths; the 30-day, 90-day and 1-year mortality are 11%, 20% and 33%, respectively (Bottle and Alylin, 2006).

Anatomy and function

The proximal femur comprises the femoral head articulating with the acetabulum as the hip joint, the femoral neck, and the greater and lesser trochanters; the latter two anatomical landmarks serve as important insertions of muscles, whose pull will cause deformity in the presence of a fracture of the neck. The proximal femur allows for the transmission of body weight from the upper body to the leg and moves the leg.

Fractures of the femoral neck are broadly divided into intracapsular or extracapsular. The hip joint capsule attaches to the pertrochanteric line anteriorly and half way up the femoral neck posteriorly. The blood supply to the femoral head is derived from an extracapsular arterial ring formed by the lateral and medial femoral circumflex arteries, the latter being dominant. Ascending branches penetrate the capsule at the intertrochanteric line forming retinacular arteries. The proximity of these retinacular vessels to the femoral neck put them at risk in femoral neck fractures (*Figure 18.1*). The blood supply to the femoral head is more abundant on the posterior aspect of the femoral neck. Knowledge

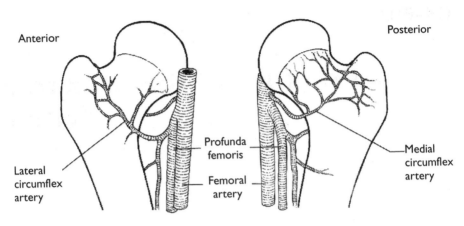

Figure 18.1. Diagrammatic representation of the arterial supply to the femoral head.

of the vascular supply in relation to fractures in this region is important as it helps in the prediction of associated complications, non-union and avascular necrosis. For practical purposes the femoral head is at significant risk of being rendered avascular by displaced intracapsular fractures.

Mechanism of injury

Fractures of the proximal femur (neck of femur fractures) are common in the elderly where the mechanism is from a simple low energy fall onto the affected hip. Less commonly fractures of the proximal femur can occur in a younger age group. These are the result of a high-energy trauma, a direct force along the femoral shaft, eg. from a road traffic accident, or a fall from a height. The greater the force dissipation the more soft tissue stripping and comminution that occurs.

Clinical picture and investigations

The patient presents with pain in the affected groin or hip and has a shortened externally rotated lower limb. The latter deformity is a result of the direction of the muscle pull on the affected bone fragments.

Elderly patients who sustain proximal femoral fractures generally have significant comorbidity and may be taking several medications, either of which may have contributed to the fall. When taking a history from the patient it should be ascertained whether the patient sustained a mechanical fall or whether there was an underlying cardiac event or blackout that precipitated the patient's collapse and fall. The patients' premorbid mobility status, ability to perform activities of daily living and social circumstances

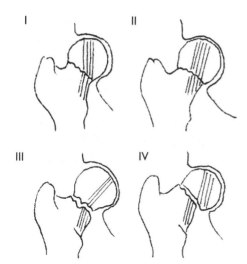

I   II

III   IV

Figure 18.2. Diagrammatic representation of Garden's classification. (Lines superimposed on the proximal femur represent the bony trabeculae.)

should be noted as the goals of treatment are to return the patient to premorbid activity levels.

Young patients who present as a result of high-energy trauma should be assessed according to Advanced Trauma Life Support (ATLS) guidelines.

Investigations which are required to diagnose the fracture are appropriate radiographs – anteroposterior (AP) pelvis and a lateral radiograph of the affected hip. In some cases if symptoms and examination findings suggest a fracture, but it is not obvious on the initial radiographs, an AP view of the involved hip with the leg maximally internally rotated to eliminate femoral anteversion is required. In 10% of cases the diagnosis is delayed. In patients where a fracture is not obvious on plain radiographs further imaging with computed tomography or magnetic resonance imaging may be indicated. Patients with radiographic evidence of osteoarthritis are highly unlikely to have sustained an intracapsular fracture as a result of the underlying joint stiffness. These patients sustain extracapsular fractures or just exacerbate their arthritic symptoms following the fall.

Other investigations that should be requested are routine blood investigations (full blood count and blood biochemistry), a chest radiograph and electrocardiogram.

Classification

Fractures of the proximal femur are generally classified as either intracapsular or extracapsular. Intracapsular fractures are classified according to Garden (1961) (*Figure 18.2*). This is based on the displacement of the trabeculae within the femoral head in relation to those in the acetabulum:

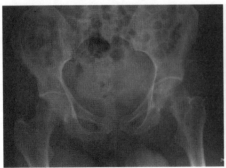

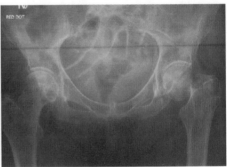

Figure 18.3. Anteroposterior pelvis radiograph showing Garden I fracture of the left neck of femur.

Figure 18.4. Anteroposterior pelvis radiograph showing Garden III fracture of the left neck of femur.

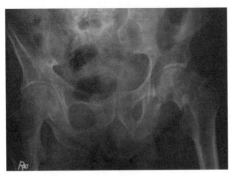

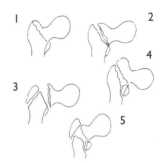

Figure 18.5. Anteroposterior pelvis radiograph showing Garden IV fracture left neck of femur.

Figure 18.6. Jensen classification of extracapsular fractures.

- I: Undisplaced valgus impaction fracture, trabecular angle >160° (*Figure 18.3*).
- II: Undisplaced fracture with no impaction (the trabeculae maintain their normal alignment).
- III: Displaced fracture where the head rotates, trabecular angle <160° (*Figure 18.4*).
- IV: Displaced fracture with no cortical contact but no rotation to the head. Trabeculae maintain normal alignment (*Figure 18.5*).

For clinical purposes and management options the grading is simplified into either undisplaced (Garden I and II) or displaced (Garden III and IV).

Extracapsular (intertrochanteric) fractures were classified by Jensen and Michaelsen (1975) into the number of fracture parts (*Figure 18.6*).

- Type 1: Undisplaced two-part fracture.

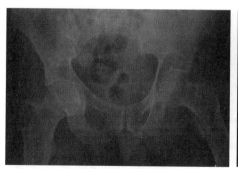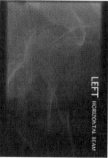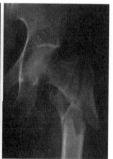

Figure 18.7. Anteroposterior pelvis radiograph showing a type 4 fracture.

Figure 18.8. Anteroposterior and lateral radiograph left hip showing four-part extracapsular fracture (type 5).

- Type 2: Displaced two-part fracture.
- Type 3: Three-part fracture, with loss of posterolateral support.
- Type 4: Three-part fracture, with loss of medial support (*Figure 18.7*).
- Type 5: Four-part fracture (*Figure 18.8*).

Management

Initial

Initial management of these injuries involves providing the patient with appropriate analgesia and intravenous fluids. Elderly patients have frequently been lying where they fell for several hours before being able to summon help, and are therefore in need of judicious fluid resuscitation. Usually bed rest is sufficient until definitive management is arranged. Occasionally application of skin traction with a 5lb weight attached is required for help with pain relief.

Definitive

Definitive care for these fractures is operative to allow early mobilisation. In the elderly group care must be taken to optimise the patient's general medical status preoperatively. There is now irrefutable evidence to support reduction and fixation of all femoral neck fractures within 24 hours of admission (Bottle and Alylin, 2006). Serious medical conditions should be maximally stabilised for at least 24 hours and pulmonary and physical therapy instituted before scheduling open surgical procedures (Jensen and Michaelsen, 1975).

Undisplaced intracapsular fractures are fixed in situ to prevent fracture displacement. This can either be achieved with cannulated hip screws (*Figure 18.9*) placed in parallel or a sliding hip screw.

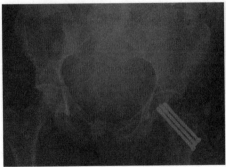 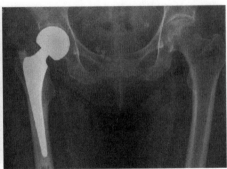

Figure 18.9. Anteroposterior pelvis radiograph showing internal fixation of left intracapsular fracture with parallel cannulated screws.

Figure 18.10. Anteroposterior pelvis radiograph showing right hip hemiarthroplasty.

Displaced intracapsular fractures have a high risk of developing avascular necrosis of the femoral head secondary to disruption of the retinacular blood vessels. The treatment of these injuries in patients over 60 years of age tends to be based on the patient's physiological age as opposed to chronological age. Options are reduction and internal fixation or arthroplasty (either total, hemi or bipolar; *Figure 18.10*). Arthroplasty has been shown to reduce the risk of revision surgery but is associated with a greater mortality risk (British Orthopaedic Association, 2003).

In the young age group who sustain an intracapsular fracture as a result of high-energy trauma the treatment, whether the fracture is undisplaced or displaced, is reduction and internal fixation. In the past this has been regarded as a surgical emergency with an aim to reduce and fix the displaced fracture as soon as possible following injury to reduce the risk of avascular necrosis developing. More recently literature has shown that although there is a decreased rate of radiographical signs of avascular necrosis, if displaced subcapital fractures are reduced and fixed within 12 hours it does not significantly affect the functional outcome (Jain *et al*, 2002).

Extracapsular fractures are treated by closed reduction of the fracture and fixation with a sliding hip screw (*Figure 18.11*) or intramedullary hip screw (*Figure 18.12*). The sliding nature of these devices allows the fracture to impact, with mobilisation, and achieves stability and union.

All methods of treatment allow for early mobilisation of the patient thus preventing the complications associated with prolonged bed rest.

Conclusion

Fractures of the neck of femur are very common in the elderly. They usually occur as a result of a low-energy fall. The blood supply to the femoral head

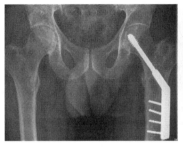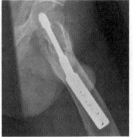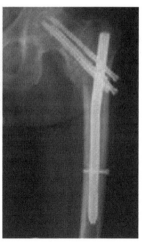

Figure 18.11. (above left and centre) Anteroposterior pelvis and lateral radiograph showing sliding hip screw fixation of left extracapsular fracture.
Figure 18.12. (right) Anteroposterior radiograph of intramedullary hip screw fixation of pertrochanteric fracture.

may be compromised due to the fracture and treatment should reflect this. Despite prompt treatment, this injury is still associated with a high incidence of complications, both medical and surgical and every effort should be made to optimise the patient pre-operatively, carry out surgery within 24 hours of admission and mobilise the patient early to minimise morbidity and mortality.

Key points

- Fractures of the neck of femur are common injuries in the elderly as a result of simple falls.
- Knowledge of the anatomy and blood supply to the proximal femur leads to a simple classification into intracapsular or extracapsular injuries, which then can lead to an algorithm for treatment options.
- Intracapsular fractures are fixed in situ if undisplaced or treated with an arthroplasty if displaced.
- Extracapsular fractures are reduced and fixed.

References

Bottle A, Alylin P (2006) Mortality associated with delay in operation after hip fracture: observational study. *Brit Med J* **332(7547)**: 947–51

British Orthopaedic Association (2003) *The Care of Fragility Fracture Patients.* British Orthopaedic Association, London

Garden RS (1961) Low-angle fixation in fractures of the femoral neck. *J Bone Joint Surg* **43-B**: 647–63

Jain R, Koo M, Kreider HJ, Schemitsch EH, Davey JR, Mahomed NL (2002) Comparison of early and delayed fixation of subcapital hip fracture in patients sixty years of age or less. *J Bone Joint Surg* **84**-**A**: 1605–12

Jensen JS, Michaelsen M (1975) Trochanteric femoral fractures treated with McLaughlin osteosynthesis. *Acta Orthop Scand* **46**: 795–803

NICE (2005) *The Clinical Effectiveness and Cost Effectiveness of Technologies for the Secondary Prevention of Osteoporotic Fractures in Postmenopausal Women.* National Institute for Clinical Excellence and Health, London

Further reading

Bhandari M, Devereaux PJ, Swiontkowski MF *et al* (2003) Internal fixation compared with arthroplasty for displaced fractures of the femoral neck. A meta analysis. *J Bone Joint Surg* **85**-**A**: 1673–81

Kenzora JE, McCarthy RE, Lowell JD, Sledge CB (1984) Hip fracture mortality. Relation to age, treatment, preoperative illness, time of surgery, and complications. *Clin Orthop Relat Res* **186**: 45–56

Parker MJ, Pryor GA, Thorngren K (1997) *Handbook of Hip Fracture Surgery.* Butterworth Heinemann, Oxford

CHAPTER 19

Femoral shaft fracture

Claire Young and Fares Haddad

Introduction

The incidence of femoral shaft fractures among an adult population has been quoted as 9.9 per 100 000 person-years (Salminen *et al*, 2000). The injury is more common in young males and the vast majority occur as a result of high-energy trauma. The osteoporotic female over 75 years of age remains a significant group sustaining this type of injury, typically from low-energy falls. Fractures of the middle third of the diaphysis seem to be the most frequent. Initial treatment proceeds with Advanced Trauma Life Support (ATLS) protocols and it must be born in mind that a fracture of the femoral diaphysis can bleed in excess of 1500ml. Therefore, aggressive resuscitation and rapid reduction and immobilisation of the grossly displaced fracture can be effective measures to treat hypovolaemic shock.

Anatomy and function

The femur is a long bone that extends from the hip to the knee. At its proximal end is the head, neck, and greater and lesser trochanters, at the distal end a metaphyseal flare to the medial and lateral condyles. The femoral diaphysis (shaft) is bowed anteriorly. The femur is a tubular bone, which gives it strength to withstand axial loading; this enables it to perform its main function of allowing standing and walking.

Muscle attachments to the femur dictate deformities of bone fragments following fractures (*Figure 19.1*). Gluteus medius and minimus attach to the greater trochanter and lead to abduction of the proximal fragment when there is a fracture distal to their insertion. The iliopsoas tendon is attached to the lesser trochanter, which causes flexion of the proximal fragment when the femur fractures below this area. The two heads of gastrocnemius (medial and lateral) take origin from the metaphyseal flare of the posterosuperior aspect of the femoral condyles; they cause flexion of the distal fragment in distal third fractures. The adductor muscles attached to the medial aspect of the femur cause an adduction deformity of the distal fragment.

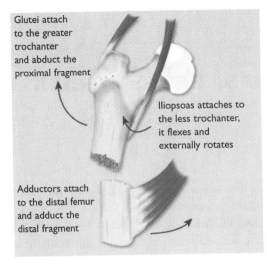

Glutei attach to the greater trochanter and abduct the proximal fragment

Iliopsoas attaches to the less trochanter, it flexes and externally rotates

Adductors attach to the distal femur and adduct the distal fragment

Figure 19.1. Diagrammatic representation of muscle attachments and direction of fracture displacement.

Mechanism of injury

Fractures of the femoral diaphysis result from major trauma, eg. road traffic accidents or falls from a height, usually a direct blow or axial loading. In the elderly, with osteoporotic bone, they can result from rotational forces, which lead to spiral fractures. Comminution of the bone is a result of the amount of energy absorbed by the bone from the impact.

Clinical picture and investigations

A femoral shaft fracture presents with pain, limb shortening, swelling and deformity. Common associated injuries are pelvic injuries, femoral neck fractures, hip dislocations, knee ligament injuries and multiple injuries. Ipsilateral femoral injuries are frequently missed and need to be specifically excluded. Neurovascular injuries associated with a diaphyseal femoral fracture are rare; however, neurovascular examination of the limb is mandatory before and after limb immobilisation. If distal pulses are not palpable then the peripheral pulses need to be assessed with a Doppler.

Associated injuries are common when major trauma is involved. These patients should be assessed using ATLS guidelines. Priority is placed on ABCs: assess the patency of the patient's airway while immobilising the cervical spine appropriately (A), check that the patient is breathing and administer oxygen via a rebreathing mask (B), and assess the patient's circulation (pulse and blood pressure) and administer intravenous fluids (C).

Radiographical evaluation should include an anteroposterior (AP) view of the pelvis, AP and lateral views of the ipsilateral hip and knee and the entire femur. Care must be taken that any immobilisation device does not obscure the bone, especially the femoral neck, leading to an associated fracture being overlooked.

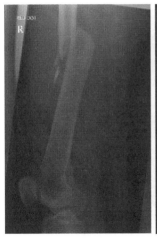 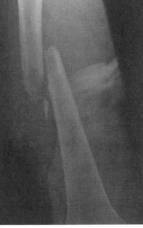

Figure 19.2. Anteroposterior and lateral radiographs showing comminuted short oblique fracture of the mid-shaft of the right femur. There is adduction and flexion of the distal fragment, shortening and medial translation of 100% of the diaphyseal diameter.

Classification

Femoral shaft fractures are classified by description:

- The status of the soft tissues – open or closed.
- Geographical location – proximal, middle or distal third.
- Fracture geometry – transverse, oblique, spiral, segmental.
- Comminution (*Figure 19.2*).
- Shortening, angulation, translation or rotatory deformity.
- Associated injuries, is it an isolated fracture or one of multiple injuries?

Management

Initial

Administer adequate analgesia to the patient. Fracture immobilisation or initial stabilisation is achieved by applying a Thomas splint (*see below*). This usually helps with pain control. Patients who sustain femoral shaft fractures can lose up to 2 litres of blood into the thigh and therefore need to receive appropriate fluid resuscitation. Immediate referral to the orthopaedic team is advised.

Definitive

Femoral diaphyseal fractures are usually displaced as a result of the significant muscle forces exerted on the fracture fragments. Operative treatment is therefore required to reduce and maintain fracture reduction and allow early mobilisation of the patient.

Methods of fixation range from plate fixation, intramedullary nailing

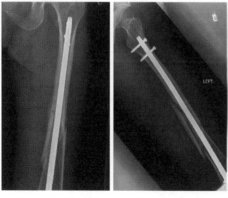

Figure 19.3. Anteroposterior and lateral radiographs showing intramedullary nail fixation of left femoral shaft fracture.

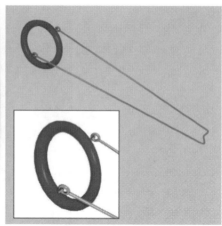

Figure 19.4. A Thomas splint.

and external fixation. The application of an external fixator to a femoral shaft fracture requires inserting the fixator pins through a large muscle bulk and pin tracks are then more prone to infections. However, 'damage control orthopaedics' as it is now referred to, has been shown to be a very effective method to treat these injuries initially. Timely definitive fixation can then be planned when the patient is optimised. Outcome has been shown to be unaffected (Harwood *et al*, 2006). Intramedullary nail fixation is more often the treatment of choice in an adult. Following closed reduction on a traction table a nail can be inserted by a relatively percutaneous approach through the piriformis fossa at the greater trochanter and statically or dynamically locked depending on the fracture configuration. An intramedullary device is more biomechanically stable compared to plate fixation and will enable immediate weight bearing (*Figure 19.3*). Pulmonary embolus, exacerbation of a pre-existing or injury related (ARDS) respiratory condition is well documented with regard to intramedullary nail insertion.

In immature patients who sustain femoral diaphyseal fractures standard nailing techniques are contraindicated as they breach the trochanteric physis, and thus have the potential for growth arrest. In children under 5 years of age conservative management with a Thomas splint or hip spica cast until fracture union is the treatment of choice. In those patients over the age of 5 years retrograde flexible nailing can be performed, avoiding the distal femoral physis, to allow early mobilisation.

Application of a Thomas splint

A Thomas splint (*Figure 19.4*) uses the principle of fixed traction with counter traction being applied against the perineum by the proximal ring to

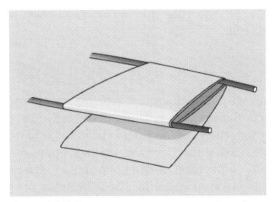

Figure 19.5. Diagrammatic representation of calico sling preparation of Thomas splint.

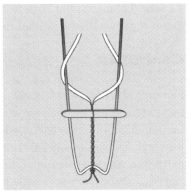

Figure 19.6. Application of traction cord to Thomas splint.

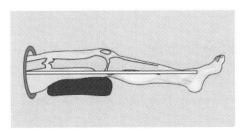

Figure 19.7. Placing a pad beneath the distal femoral fragment corrects flexion deformity.

maintain femoral fracture reduction. It will not reduce the fracture; this must be achieved before splint application by manipulation. Splints come in different sizes. To select the correct size the circumference of the thigh needs to be measured. This is difficult to achieve on the injured side and therefore the uninjured side is measured and 5cm added to this, allowing for swelling (the ring should fit the thigh as snugly as possible without causing skin irritation). The splint is prepared by placing sheets of calico bandaging over the metal sides as slings (*Figure 19.5*), cotton wool padding is then used on top of this. The splint is then carefully placed under the affected limb.

Skin traction is applied to the leg from the distal femur to the ankles, taking care that the padding protects the malleoli. The traction is then wrapped around the sides of the splint winding the medial cord from inside to out and the lateral cord from outside to in (*Figure 19.6*). The cords are then crossed and tied to the distal end of the splint. Sufficient tension is added to the traction by winding the cord over two tongue depressors (two are used to prevent the depressor from breaking with the strain). Following splint application the distal neurovascular status of the limb should be reassessed. The distal fracture fragment tends to flex because of the pull of the gastrocnemius. This backward angulation can be corrected by placing a large pad behind the distal fragment to act as a fulcrum (*Figure 19.7*).

Further radiographs are taken of the femur in the splint to ascertain appropriate fracture reduction has been achieved.

The Thomas splint then needs to be suspended from an overhead beam so that it moves with the patient in the bed.

Conclusion

Femoral shaft fractures occur frequently in high-energy trauma such as road traffic accidents or falls from a height. Standard resuscitation techniques must be implemented initially, followed by reduction and temporary stabilisation of the fracture. Associated injuries must be looked for. Once the patient is optimised, definitive surgical treatment, usually in the form of an intramedullary device, can be carried out. A multi-discliplinary approach to management is often required from the outset.

Key points

- ####s tend to result from high energy trauma.
- Advanced Trauma Life Support principles should be applied in initial patient management.
- Thomas splint application gives initial temporary fracture stabilisation and aids pain control.
- Definitive fracture management is operative by intramedullary nail fixation.

References

Harwood PJ, Giannoudis PV, Probst C, Kettek C, Pape HC (2006) The risk of local infective complications after damage control procedures for femoral shaft fracture. *J Orthop Trauma* **20(3)**:181–9

Salminen ST, Pihlajamaki HK, Avikainen VJ, Bostman OM (2000) Population based epidemiologic and morphologic study of femoral shaft fractures. *Clin Orthop Relat Res* **372**: 241–9

Further reading

Charnley J (1999) Fractures of the shaft of the femur. In: *The Closed Treatment of Common Fractures*. Golden Jubilee Edition. Colt Books, Cambridge: 166–96

CHAPTER 20

Fractures around the knee

Claire Young and Fares Haddad

Introduction

Most fractures around the knee mainly involve either the tibial plateau or the distal femur. The anatomy mechanism of injury and treatment for each is vastly different. The severity of a tibial plateau fracture and the complexity of its treatment depend on the energy imparted to the limb. Low-energy injuries typically cause unilateral depression-type fractures, whereas high-energy injuries can lead to comminuted fractures with significant osseous, soft-tissue, and neurovascular injury. Distal femoral fractures account for 4–7% of all femoral fractures and are usually the result of injury to the knee in a flexed position. Both types of injury may involve the joint surface and thus anatomical reduction is mandatory.

Tibial plateau

Anatomy and function

The proximal tibia forms the distal surface of the knee joint. The medial plateau is larger and concave anteroposteriorly and mediolaterally. The lateral plateau is smaller, higher and convex in both anteroposterior and mediolateral directions. The central non-articular area comprises the tibial spines with the anterior cruciate ligament taking origin from the anterior spine.

The medial plateau is stronger than the lateral and injuries to the medial side are frequently associated with significant soft tissue trauma as they result from more violent injuries.

Mechanism of injury

Fractures of the tibial plateau have a bimodal distribution. In the younger age group they result from high-energy trauma or falls from a height. The second group occur in the elderly with more osteoporotic bone. Fractures occur from varus or valgus directed forces, axial compression or a combination of both. Shearing or compressive forces from the femoral condyles result in split or depression fractures.

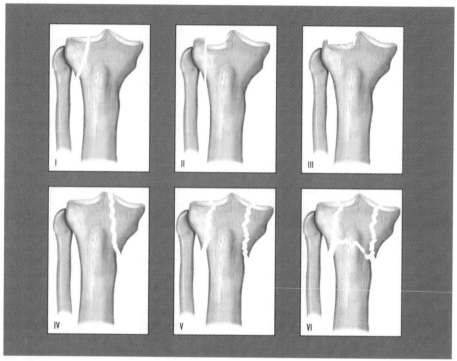

Figure 20.1. Diagrammatic representation of Schatzker's classification of tibial plateau fractures.

Clinical picture and investigations

Evaluation of the patient begins with a careful history. Any patient who has sustained a significant fall must be assumed to have other injuries until proven otherwise.

The patient complains of pain, swelling of the knee as a result of a haemarthrosis and inability to weight-bear on the affected side.

Having been administered appropriate analgesia the patient is examined. Careful evaluation of the soft tissue envelope must be performed. As tibial plateau fractures following significant trauma may be associated with a knee dislocation at the time of impact, which then relocates, the neurological and vascular status of the limb should be carefully assessed. Particular attention should be made to assessing the function of the common peroneal nerve (ankle and toe dorsiflexion and sensation over the first web space). Joint stability is assessed by examination of the collateral ligaments and cruciate ligaments. This may be difficult with the patient awake and can be subsequently performed under anaesthesia.

Radiographs of the knee, both anteroposterior and lateral views, may not confirm the injury. Oblique view radiographs are often helpful in evaluating the nature of the injury in these cases.

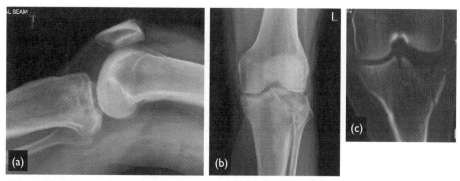

Figure 20.2. Schatzker II fracture of the left tibial plateau. (a) Lateral radiograph. (b) Anteroposterior radiograph. Note double shadow of articular surface on lateral radiograph (remember that the lateral plateau should be higher than the medial). (c) Coronal computed tomography slice showing split depression.

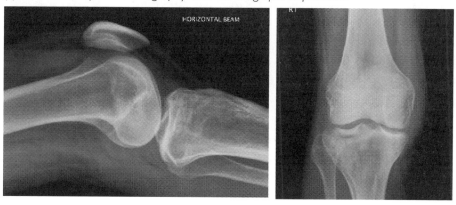

Figure 20.3. Anteroposterior and lateral radiographs showing Schatzker III fracture right tibial plateau.

The presence and location of a fracture with the degree of displacement and any joint surface depression is noted.

Classification

Tibial plateau fractures are commonly classified according to Schatzker and McBroom (1979) (*Figure 20.1*):

- I: A split fracture of the lateral plateau
- II: A split depression fracture of the lateral plateau (*Figure 20.2*)
- III: A pure depression fracture of the lateral plateau (*Figure 20.3*)
- IV: A medial plateau fracture (*Figure 20.4*).
- V: A bicondylar fracture with metaphyseal continuity.
- VI: A bicondylar fracture with metaphyseal–diaphyseal discontinuity.

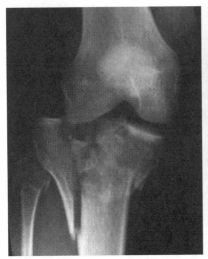

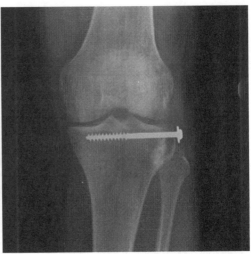

Figure 20.4. Anteroposterior
radiograph showing Schatzker VI
fracture of the right tibial plateau.

Figure 20.5. Anteroposterior radiograph
showing percutaneous screw. Fixation of
Schatzker I fracture of the left tibial plateau.

Management

Initial
Initial management is splintage of the knee, usually with an above-knee backslab
that incorporates medial and lateral support around the knee to prevent rotation.
These fractures are articular injuries and usually require operative intervention,
as definitive management, to restore the congruity of the articular surface.

It is often difficult to fully assess the nature and configuration of the
fracture from plain radiographs and the patient should be further evaluated with
computed tomography (CT) (*Figure 20.2*).

Definitive
If the fracture is undisplaced, there is no articular fragment depression or there
is limited displacement and/or depression then non-operative management
of the fracture with a cast brace is appropriate. This allows for early joint
movement to prevent stiffness but the patient remains non-weight-bearing
initially. Weekly radiographs are required in the first few weeks to ensure that
the fracture position is maintained.

Those patients with displaced fractures or depression of the articular surface
require operative fracture reduction and fixation. Failure to restore bony anatomy
and ligament function results in joint instability. This can be achieved by a variety
of different methods; the decision is made based on the degree of bony deformity
and the associated soft tissue injury. Options range from elevation of the joint
surface and holding with percutaneous screws (*Figure 20.5*), arthroscopic-

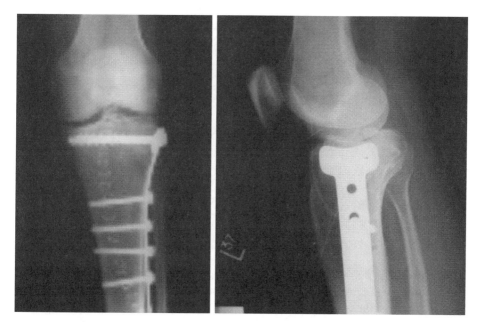

Figure 20.6. Anteroposterior and lateral radiographs of buttress plating of a Schatzker II fracture.

assisted surgery, bone grafting, buttress plating (*Figure 20.6*) or circular frame external fixation.

Distal femur

Anatomy and function

The distal femur is divided into a supracondylar and intercondylar area. The distal femur flares in its metaphyseal region into two condyles. Anteriorly the articular surface has a depression, the trochlear groove, for patellofemoral articulation. Posteriorly is the intercondylar notch. At the maximum flare medially is the adductor tubercle. In the sagittal plane the femoral shaft is aligned with the anterior half of the condyles.

Mechanism of injury

Injuries to the distal femur occur in the young age group as a result of high-energy trauma caused by a direct load on the flexed knee. These are frequently open and highly comminuted injuries and associated injuries must be excluded (eg. ipsilateral acetabular fractures, hip dislocation, femoral neck or shaft fracture). In the elderly this injury is the result of low energy trauma, such as a simple fall on the flexed knee.

Clinical picture and investigations

The patient usually presents with a painful, swollen knee secondary to a haemarthrosis and inability to move the limb. Initial management involves taking a careful history; in the case of high-energy injuries the patient should be managed following Advanced Trauma Life Support (ATLS) guidelines. Careful evaluation of the distal neurovascular status of the limb should be performed. The patient should be administered appropriate analgesia and the affected limb splinted with an above-knee plaster backslab while applying gentle in-line traction to the leg to help to reduce the fracture. Diagnosis is made from appropriate anteroposterior and lateral radiographs of the knee and distal femur.

Classification

Fractures are either an extra-articular supracondylar fracture or intra-articular intercondylar fracture, displaced or undisplaced.

Owing to the muscle forces on the fracture fragments supracondylar fractures tend to shorten with posterior angulation and displacement of the distal fragment secondary to the pull of the two heads of gastrocnemius. Intracondylar fractures are associated with malrotation of the fragments.

These fractures are classified according to the AO system described by Muller *et al* (1979) (*Figure 20.7*):

- Type A: Extra-articular fractures (*Figure 20.8*).
- Type B: Partial articular fractures (unicondylar).
- Type C: Bicondylar fractures.

Management

Initial
Administer adequate analgesia to the patient before splinting the leg in an above-knee backslab, with a plaster backshell and U slab to allow for rotational stability of the knee. Assess the distal neurovascular status of the limb following reduction and immobilising the fracture.

Definitive
The aim of further treatment is to restore length, rotation, axial alignment and articular congruency.

Undisplaced fractures can be treated non-operatively with a cast brace, which allows for early controlled knee movement. Regular radiographs are required to ascertain that fracture position is maintained.

Operative intervention is indicated for displaced intra-articular fractures,

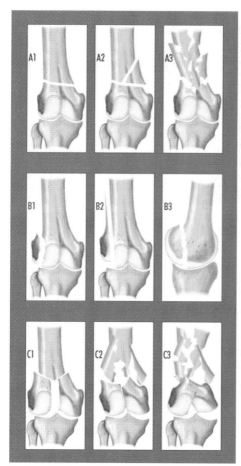

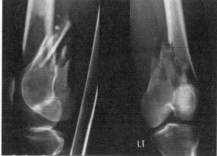

Figure 20.8. Anteroposterior and lateral radiographs of type A fracture left distal femur.

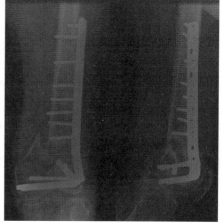

Figure 20.9. Anteroposterior and lateral radiographs of supracondylar nail fixation of type A fracture.

Figure 20.7. Diagrammatic representation of distal femoral fractures.

open fractures, fractures with associated vascular compromise, in association with ipsilateral tibial fractures and in polytrauma cases. A better functional result and fewer complications are achieved following open reduction and internal fixation even in the elderly group (Butt *et al*, 1995). Methods of internal fixation are either supracondylar nailing (*Figure 20.9*), angled fixation devices (dynamic condylar screw) (*Figure 20.10*) or LISS (less invasive skeletal stabilisation) plating.

Conclusion

Fractures around the knee can be intra-articular or extra-articular. The former will require operative anatomical reduction in a significant proportion of cases. If knee dislocation is suspected, careful vascular assessment is required. Significant soft-tissue and ligamentous injury is frequent with both types of fracture and may

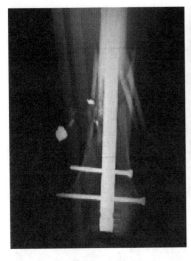

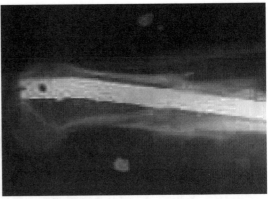

Figure 20.10. Anteroposterior and lateral radiographs showing dynamic condylar screw fixation of left distal femoral fracture.

only be apparent some time after the injury or when the patient is examined under anaesthesia. Acute management should follow ATLS guidelines and plaster of Paris immobilisation is satisfactory treatment initially.

Key points

- Fractures around the knee in the young patient are a result of high-energy trauma.
- Patients present with painful, swollen knees after injury and are unable to weight-bear.
- Initial management involves Advanced Trauma Life Support principles, analgesia and splinting of the limb.
- The key to definitive management is restoring the congruity of the joint surface which usually requires operative intervention.

References

Butt MS, Krikler SR, Ali MS (1995) Displaced fractures of the distal femur in elderly patients. *J Bone Joint Surg* **77-B**: 110–14

Muller MG, Allgöwer M, Schneider R, Willenegger H (1979) *Manual of Internal Fixation.* Springer Verlag, New York

Schatzker J, McBroom R (1979) Tibial plateau fractures. The Toronto experience 1968–1975. *Clin Orthop* **138**: 94–104

CHAPTER 21

Soft tissue knee injuries

Rahul Patel and Fares Haddad

Introduction

The knee is the most commonly injured joint in sport and exercise, and soccer and skiing carry the highest risk (Nicholl *et al*, 1991). In the largest study of its kind, 39.8% of all athletic injuries were related to the knee joint. Injuries were more common in males and almost 50% of the patients were between the ages of 20–29 years at the time of injury (Majewski *et al*, 2006). Knee injuries can result from contact and non-contact mechanisms. The resulting lesions may be isolated, combined, partial or complete and may be associated with bony injuries.

Anatomy and function

The knee is the largest joint in body. It is a synovial joint of the modified hinge (condyloid) type between the distal end of the femur, the patella and the proximal end of the tibia. The femoral articular surface is formed of three surfaces: a middle concave surface for the patella (trochlea), and medial and lateral condylar surfaces for the tibia which are markedly convex. The upper surface of each tibia is oval and slightly concave. See *Figure 21.1*.

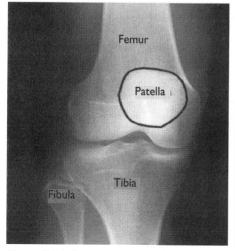 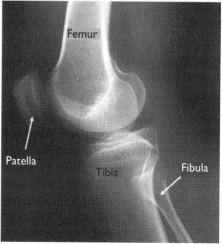

Figure 21.1. Bony anatomy of the knee joint. Anteroposterior and lateral radiographs.

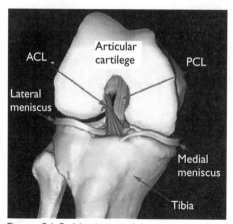

Figure 21.2. Menisci and cruciate ligaments.

The capsule is attached to bone near the margins of the articular surfaces. The patellar tendon extends from the apex of the patella to the tibial tuberosity. There are two collateral ligaments on either side of the knee: the medial collateral ligament (MCL) is a broad flat band originating from the femur and inserting into the proximal tibial metaphysis (Gerdy's tubercle) and has attachments to the capsule. The lateral collateral ligament is a rounded cord originating from the lateral femur extending to the head of fibula and is distinctly separate from the capsule.

The anterior cruciate ligament (ACL) runs upwards, backwards and laterally from the tibial spines to the medial surface of the lateral femoral condyle. Its function is to prevent anterior translation of tibia on femur but also provides rotatory stability.

The posterior cruciate ligament (PCL) runs forwards, upwards and medially from the back of the intercondylar notch of the tibia to the lateral surface of the medial femoral condyle. It prevents the tibia sagging back on the femur and also provides rotatory stability.

The menisci are two crescentic pieces of fibrocartilage with thickened outer margins. Each lies on a tibial condyle with its ends (anterior and posterior horns) attached to the intercondylar region and the outer margin attached to capsule. The medial meniscus is larger and semi-circular. The lateral meniscus is smaller and is C-shaped. The lateral meniscus is separated by capsule posteriorly so is more mobile than the medial meniscus. See *Figure 21.2*. Their primary function is to contribute to load distribution and improve stability of the knee joint.

The knee is capable of flexion, extension and rotation. Flexion occurs as a result of hamstring action, aided by gastrocnemius; the range of motion is restricted by apposition of the surfaces of the calf and thigh. Extension is a function of the quadriceps and iliotibial tract muscles. A small amount of medial rotation and lateral rotation is produced by hamstrings when the knee is flexed to 90°. The femoral condyles roll back on the tibial condyles during flexion and the capsular and cruciate ligaments become taut when the leg is nearly straight.

Mechanisms of injury and clinical findings

When considering mechanisms of soft tissue injury to the knee it is most appropriate to discuss this by particular anatomical structure including clinical

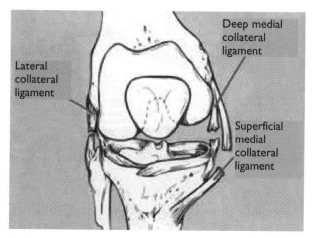

Figure 21.3 Medial collateral ligament rupture.

findings. However, most mechanisms will be responsible for a sequence of injury, involving multiple structures at their most severe. This must be borne in mind when examining the knee joint for soft tissue injury.

The first examining doctor is often fortunate to assess a soft tissue knee injury in its acute stages, and may be able to collect vital information. The history is fresh in the patient's mind and may be of considerable value in determining the diagnosis. Moreover, some signs and symptoms may be more easily gleaned before swelling, bruising and pain inhibition set in. In every case the assessment should include an examination of both knees as well as an assessment of the hip and ankle on the affected side. A neurovascular assessment is mandatory. The examiner is almost always fortunate in having the contralateral limb for comparison.

Collateral ligament injuries

The patient reports a history of twisting or wrenching the knee. The injury commonly occurs while the knee is flexed. Occasionally a pop is heard or felt but this does not necessarily imply an anterior cruciate ligament tear.

Medial collateral ligament (MCL) injuries (*Figure 21.3*) are much more common. Look for bruising and feel for medial tenderness above or below the joint line. The knee should be stressed into valgus firstly with the knee extended, and then with the knee held in 30° of flexion. If the knee opens up in full extension, several ligaments have been injured, the extremity must be assessed for a vascular injury and immediate orthopaedic referral is required.

The lateral collateral ligament (LCL) complex is more rarely injured. The knee joint opens up with varus stress. Always assess for associated injuries and look for a foot-drop as the common peroneal nerve may be injured.

X-rays are mandatory to exclude bony injuries or avulsions in both situations.

Cruciate ligament injuries

Anterior cruciate ligament (ACL) injuries account for up to 50% of documented ligamentous knee injuries (Majewski *et al*, 2006). Contrary to popular belief, ACL injuries are more commonly seen after non-contact rather than contact injuries. Patients often describe one of the following modes of injury:

- *Deceleration*. These may be seen in basketball or football players who change direction. If the lower leg is internally rotated at the time, the ACL is at risk.
- *Flexion/valgus/external rotation*. As the knee is bent and twisted out (for example if a football or rugby boot is stuck in the turf or a ski binding does not release the boot in a twisting fall), the medial knee ligaments are initially injured and then the ACL gives way. These injuries are often associated with medial meniscal tears – the so-called unhappy triad of O'Donoghue.
- *Hyperextension*. This may be seen in basketball and volleyball players who land awkwardly and in gymnasts during the dismount. It is the mechanism of injury in some footballers who cannot control their landing after going up for a header.
- A *direct blow* to the knee or shin can also lead to an ACL tear. These injuries are usually associated with damage to other structures within the knee.

In over 50% of cases, the patient will hear a 'pop' or feel tearing within the knee. The patient is usually unable to continue playing sport and the knee swells rapidly. The swelling is due to a haemarthrosis (bleeding into the joint) and 80% of patients attending accident and emergency with acute haemarthroses have sustained ACL injuries. Other causes of haemarthroses include osteochondral fractures (aspiration will reveal fat globules as well as blood) and peripheral meniscal tears.

Anteroposterior knee stability should be assessed at 20° (Lachmann) and 90° (anterior drawer test – *Figure 21.4*) flexion and compared to the other side. A positive pivot shift test is pathognomic but is difficult to perform in the acute setting because of pain inhibition.

Posterior cruciate ligament injuries require a greater force: these are more commonly direct blows to the anterior aspect of the knee (*Figure 21.5*) or severe hyperextension injuries. The initial symptoms are similar to those for ACL injuries. Examination reveals the posterior sag sign when the knee is flexed to 90° in comparison to the uninjured side. The posterior drawer test may be positive.

Plain radiographs are required in order to exclude bony avulsions for both types of injury.

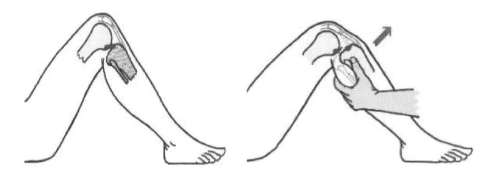

Figure 21.4. Anterior drawer test for diagnosis of anterior cruciate ligament rupture.

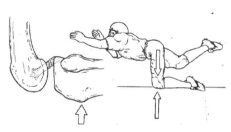

Figure 21.5. Mechanism of posterior cruciate ligament rupture.

Meniscal injuries

These injuries usually result from a rotational stress applied to a flexed, weight-bearing knee. Medial meniscus (MM) injuries are more common than lateral meniscus (LM) injuries; this is due to the fact that the MM is less mobile because of its capsular attachments. Tears cause characteristic symptoms of pain, swelling, locking and giving way. On examination, there is often an effusion, and the patient is very tender on palpation of the joint line (not above or below) and cannot squat down fully. McMurray's test (rotation of the tibia on the femoral condyles with the knee in deep flexion) may be positive (painful) if a tear exists. If the joint is rested, the symptoms usually subside, only to return with twisting or trivial straining of the joint. The knee may also give way spontaneously.

Locking (the inability to straighten the knee) can occur in certain types of tears where the displaced meniscus blocks full extension of the joint. This becomes an urgent surgical problem as the knee must not be left in a fixed flexed position. Patients with true locking are either admitted directly or referred urgently to the next available clinic.

Patellar dislocation

Many patients are predisposed to patellar dislocation through anatomical variants and poor knee biomechanics. Patellar dislocation usually results from sudden contraction of the quadriceps muscle, especially when the knee is in valgus and externally rotated, eg. when running and dodging to one side. The patella dislocates laterally and can spontaneously reduce in some cases. The patient reports the knee as having gone 'out of joint', and is left with medial knee pain above and below the joint line indicative of a medial patellar retinaculum tear rather than a meniscal or medial collateral ligament injury. If the patella remains dislocated, it can usually be easily reduced with distraction of the patient, analgesia and gentle knee extension with a medial force applied to the patella.

Radiographs are mandatory regardless of whether the patella has spontaneously relocated or not. Anteroposterior and lateral views of the knee and skyline views of the patella are required. Osteochondral fractures are managed with acute surgical intervention within a week.

Extensor apparatus failure

If the patient is unable to straight leg raise and does not have X-ray evidence of a patellar fracture, an injury to the quadriceps tendon or patellar tendon should be suspected. A gap in the affected tendon is often palpable. The mechanism of injury is usually related to a sudden deceleration of the lower leg relative to the rest of the body such as a stumble on a wet or muddy surface. These patients must be referred to the inpatient team for tendon repair.

Clinical picture and investigations

A full history must be taken, including determination of mechanism of injury, whether the patient was able to carry on participating in the activity or able to bear weight after the injury and whether the knee became swollen immediately (most probably a haemarthrosis) or over the next 24–48 hours (traumatic effusion) as this will influence suspicion of injury to particular structures. Aspiration of a haemarthrosis (*see later*) is a very effective pain-relieving measure and can be diagnostic in terms of confirming bleeding in the joint and for observation for fat globules interspersed in the blood as this evidences a fracture. If a patient is assessed primarily some days or weeks after an injury then it is important to determine weight-bearing status since the injury, whether the pain has settled and whether the knee has clicked, locked or given way.

Plain radiographs of the knee (anteroposterior and lateral views) are mandatory for all suspected soft tissue injuries, to exclude fracture and avulsion injuries. Skyline views of the patella may be requested for suspected cases of dislocation.

Magnetic resonance imaging (MRI) has become the gold standard method of detecting soft tissue injuries of the knee, but should be requested by the orthopaedic team at assessment, typically at least two weeks after injury.

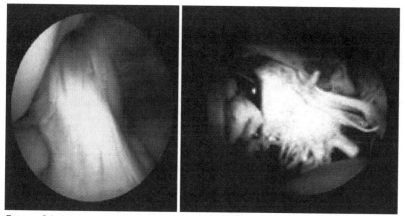

Figure 21.6 Intact (left) and ruptured (right) anterior cruciate ligament.

Management

Initial

If there is any doubt over the injury in this area, orthopaedic opinion should be sought. Interpretation of X-rays can be difficult. All fractures must be discussed with the orthopaedic team. Isolated soft tissue injuries can usually be treated acutely with rest, ice, compression and elevation (RICE). Patients should be given a brace, one which allows little or no movement if in doubt. Crutches, instructions to the patient not to bear weight and anti-inflammatory medication if suitable should also be administered. Referral to the next available clinic must be arranged for further assessment and examination as commonly, more useful clinical information can be gained from the knee joint 2–4 weeks after injury.

Definitive

Collateral ligament injuries are treated conservatively with 4–6 weeks of bracing as standard with increasing range of movement and physiotherapy thereafter.

Meniscal injuries may need MRI to confirm the diagnosis. If the tear is small, some patients have a good outcome with physiotherapy alone; if the tear is peripheral it may heal as the blood supply is good in this area. Most patients require surgical intervention in the form of an arthroscopy to remedy the problem. This can be carried out safely, non-acutely.

Cruciate ligament ruptures (*Figure 21.6*) and associated injuries (ie. meniscal and collateral ligament tears) are initially treated conservatively with bracing and physiotherapy; professional athletes may undergo surgical intervention much earlier if diagnosis is made acutely for earlier return to sport.

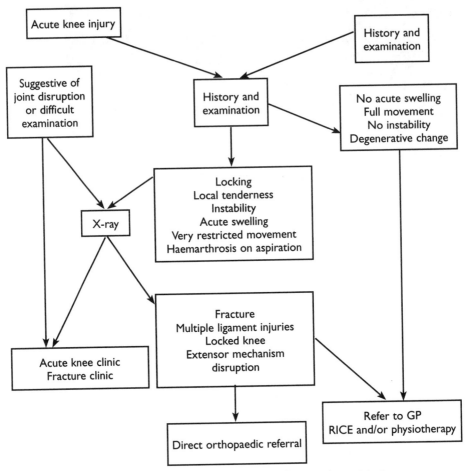

Figure 21.7 Algorithm for management of acute soft tissue knee injuries.

Decisions regarding reconstruction of the cruciate ligaments are made after a comprehensive assessment of each individual's activity level and expectations as well as age and other factors such as likelihood of compliance with an extended rehabilitation programme.

Patella dislocation must be braced at the very least in full extension for a moderate period. First time dislocations may be treated in a long leg cylinder cast for up to 10 weeks. Physiotherapy, particularly strengthening of the vastus medialis obliquus muscle, forms the mainstay of treatment.

Extensor tendon rupture almost always requires reconstruction. Diagnosis is often effectively confirmed using ultrasound.

An algorithm for management of acute soft tissue knee injuries is shown in *Figure 21.7.*

Conclusion

The history and mechanism of injury are essential information when diagnosing knee injuries. Initial treatment usually involves rest, icing, compression and elevation and expert opinion should be sought thereafter. The exceptions are soft tissue knee injuries associated with fracture and knee dislocation; these must be referred immediately. Swelling and pain inhibition limits useful clinical information being gleaned from the examination acutely and thus sequential assessment with the aid of imaging adjuncts may be required.

Key points

- The knee is the most commonly injured joint in sport and exercise, and soccer, netball and rugby carry the highest risk.
- Knee injuries can result from contact and non-contact mechanisms.
- The resulting lesions may be isolated, combined, partial or complete and may be associated with bony injuries.
- The history is of considerable value in determining the diagnosis.
- Anterior cruciate ligament injuries account for up to 50% of documented ligamentous knee injuries.
- Anterior cruciate ligament injuries are more commonly seen after non-contact rather than contact injuries.
- Other causes of haemarthroses include osteochondral fractures and peripheral meniscal tears.
- Posterior cruciate ligament injuries require a greater force: these are more commonly direct blows to the anterior aspect of the knee or severe hyperextension injuries.
- Meniscal injuries usually result from a rotational stress applied to a flexed, weight bearing knee.
- Locking (the inability to straighten the knee) can occur in certain types of tears where the displaced meniscus blocks full extension of the joint. This becomes an urgent surgical problem as the knee must not be left in a fixed flexed position.
- Plain radiographs of the knee (anterioposterior and lateral) are mandatory for all suspected soft tissue injuries, to exclude fracture and avulsion injuries.
- Isolated soft tissue injuries can usually be treated acutely with rest, ice, compression and elevation (RICE).

References

Majewski M, Susanne H, Klaus S. (2006) Epidemiology of athletic knee injuries: A 10-year study. *Knee* **13(3)**: 184–8

Nicholl JP, Coleman P, Williams BT (1991) *Injuries in Sport and Exercise*. Sports Council, London

CHAPTER 22

Tibial and fibular fractures

Claire Young and Fares Haddad

Introduction

The tibia is the commonest site of diaphyseal fracture with an incidence of approximately 2 per 10 000 population. Fractures can be open or closed, displaced or undisplaced, angulated, shortened or rotated. The degree of comminution relates to energy imparted and extent of soft tissue injury. The latter may have an effect on time to union and associated complications. This chapter addresses fractures of the shaft only.

Anatomy and function

The tibia is the main bone of the lower leg. The diaphysis is triangular in cross section with an anteriorly directed apex. The medial border of the tibia lies subcutaneously. Proximally it articulates with the distal femur at the knee joint and distally with the talus at the ankle. It allows the limb to weight bear, acts as a lever arm for the calf muscles and helps transmit the neurovascular structures to the ankle and foot.

The fibula is the lesser bone on the lateral aspect of the leg. It plays no role in the knee joint but has an important role in ankle stability. The fibula is attached to the tibia by an interosseous membrane. The common peroneal nerve winds around the neck of the fibula and is not infrequently injured in proximal fibula fractures.

The calf is divided into four compartments by intermuscular septums: anterior, lateral, deep posterior and superficial posterior. These form separate myofascial compartments each with its individual neurovascular structures (*Figure 22.1, Table 22.1*). Knowledge of these compartments is essential in the diagnosis of compartment syndrome (*see below and Chapter 4*).

Mechanism of injury

The mechanism of injury varies. It can be as simple as a fall with a twisting force or due to road traffic accidents, sports accidents (football, skiing) or crush injuries. Direct blows result in transverse fractures with or without butterfly fragments, twisting injuries cause spiral fractures. It is important to differentiate

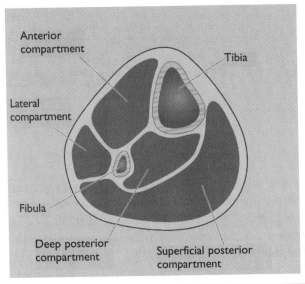

Figure 22.1. Cross-section of calf showing musculofascial compartments.

Table I. Muscle groups contained in each lower leg compartment

Compartment	Muscles	Function	Sensory distribution
Anterior	Tibialis anterior Extensor hallucis longus Extensor digitorum communis Peroneus tertius	Toe and ankle dorsiflexion	First and second dorsal web spaces (deep peroneal nerve)
Lateral	Peroneus brevis Peroneus longus	Ankle eversion	Lateral dorsum of foot (superficial peroneal nerve)
Superficial posterior	Gastrocnemius Soleus Plantaris	Ankle plantar flexion (sural nerve)	Lateral side of heel
Deep posterior	Flexor digitorum longus	Toe plantar flexion	
Sole of foot	Flexor hallucis longus Tibialis posterior	Ankle inversion	(posterior tibial nerve)

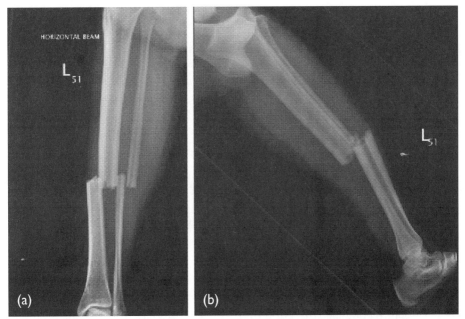

Figure 22.2. (a) Anteroposterior (AP) and (b) lateral radiographs of transverse fracture of the middle third of the left tibia. Note associated rotational deformity and knee dislocation (lateral view of ankle joint with AP view of dislocated knee joint on same film).

early between low and high-energy injuries. The former tend to be more benign and have a better prognosis than the latter which may be associated with multiple injuries sustained by the patient and have a more sinister prognosis sed on the degree of soft tissue injury sustained.

Clinical picture and investigations

Patients usually present with a history of trauma, following which they have pain in the lower leg, are unable to weight-bear, have limb instability and may or may not have a deformed limb.

Initial assessment involves determining whether it is an isolated injury or part of multiple injuries sustained by the patient. Is the injury open or closed (*see below*)? The distal neurovascular status of the limb needs to be assessed documenting the presence or absence of both the dorsalis pedis and posterior tibial pulses. If pulses are absent then Doppler assessment of flow in the vessels is required.

Anteroposterior and lateral radiographs of the limb confirm the nature of the injury. The images need to include the knee joint and the ankle joint on the same film to determine if any rotational deformity to the fracture is present (*Figure 22.2*).

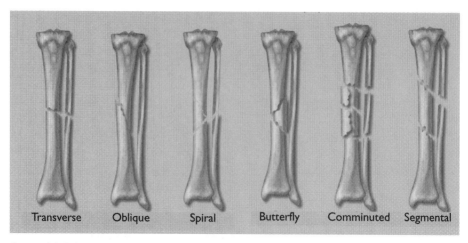

Figure 22.3. Diagrammatic representation of fracture geometry.

Classification

Tibial fractures are classified descriptively according to:

- Open or closed.
- Geographical location in bone (proximal, middle or distal third).
- Fracture geometry (transverse, oblique, spiral, segmental) (*Figure 22.3*).
- Displacement, angulation, rotational deformity of fracture fragments.

Open fractures are classified according to Gustilo and Anderson (1976):

- Grade I: A wound <1cm.
- Grade II: A wound <10cm.
- Grade III: A wound >10cm (a high energy injury, a highly contaminated wound or underlying segmental fracture).
- Grade III is subdivided into:
  - A: Adequate soft tissue coverage possible.
  - B: Massive soft tissue disruption.
  - C: Associated vascular injury.

Management

Initial
The patient requires appropriate analgesia, reduction and immobilisation of the fracture. A backslab should be applied from midthigh to toes with the knee flexed approximately 20° and the ankle at 90° to the tibia. The plaster slabs should comprise one along the back of the thigh and calf running

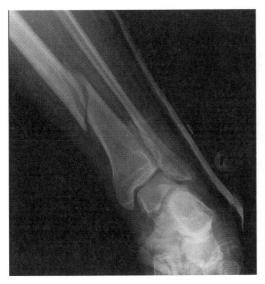

Figure 22.4. Anteroposterior radiograph of short spiral fracture of the junction of the middle/distal thirds of the left tibia.

onto the sole of the foot and one running as a U slab along both sides of the leg to give rotational stability to the splint. The patient requires further radiographs following plaster application to check the reduction of the fracture (*Figure 22.4*).

Definitive

The definitive treatment of tibial fractures depends on the fracture configuration and stability, and the condition of the surrounding soft tissue envelope. Closed fractures that are undisplaced can be treated non-operatively with an above-knee plaster for 4–6 weeks followed by a patella tendon-bearing cast or splint until fracture union. Initial weekly radiographs are taken to ensure alignment is maintained. However the length of time of non-operative treatment and its associated complications must be weighed up against those of operative treatment and early mobilisation and return to work/activity.

Indications for operative intervention are malalignment or angulation, comminution (including segmental fractures), open fractures, failed closed reduction, a multiply injured patient, an ipsilateral femoral shaft fracture, and fractures associated with compartment syndrome or vascular injuries.

Open fractures require the wound to be thoroughly debrided and lavaged to deal with the bone and soft tissue contamination followed by fracture stabilisation. The options for bony stabilisation are intramedullary nailing (*Figure 22.5*), external fixation (*Figure 22.6*) and internal plate fixation (*Figure 22.7*). Stabilisation in the presence of significant soft tissue injury would tend to involve intramedullary fixation to allow adequate access to the soft tissues for their management and any reconstructive surgery by plastic surgeons.

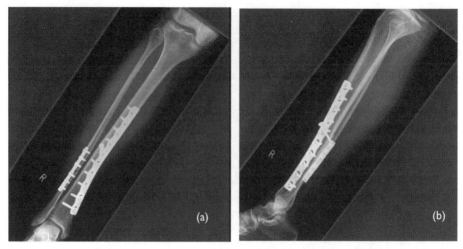

Figure 22.5. (a) Anteroposterior and (b) lateral radiographs of a locked intramedullary nail fixation of an oblique fracture of right tibia.

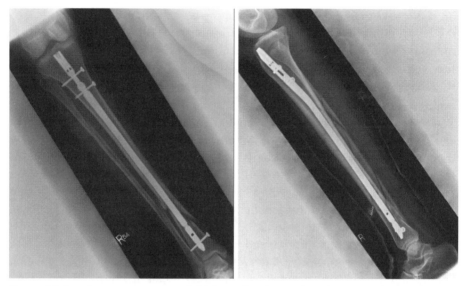

Figure 22.6. a. Anteroposterior and (b) lateral radiographs of external fixation of comminuted distal third of a tibial fracture.

Compartment syndrome

This occurs when the intracompartmental pressure rises to greater than the capillary perfusion pressure and there is failure of oxygenation of the compartment contents. The muscles of the limb are surrounded by a fascial membrane that has a finite degree of expansion. When the limb is injured or the bone fractured there is bleeding into the compartment. The compartment

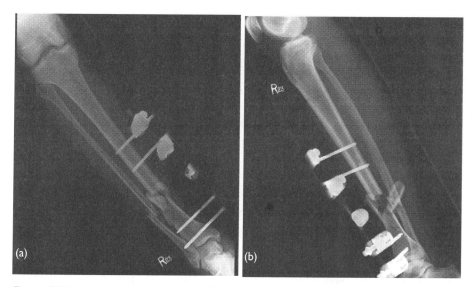

Figure 22.7. (a) Anteroposterior and (b) lateral radiographs of internal plate fixation of right tibia and fibula fractures.

can swell and expand to its maximum volume causing pain but still allowing adequate capillary perfusion of its contents. Any additional swelling will cause the intracompartmental pressure to rise, as it can no longer expand. This initially blocks venous drainage from the compartment, which only exacerbates the volume problem and leads to a further rise in intracompartmental pressure until it exceeds capillary filling pressure and oxygenation of the tissues ceases.

Compartment syndrome presents with pain out of proportion to the injury sustained. There is increased pain on passive stretching of the muscles in the involved compartment. By the time the patient has signs of reduced capillary refill, loss of palpable pulses and paraesthesia in the limb muscle necrosis has undoubtedly already commenced.

Compartment syndrome is a clinical diagnosis. Intracompartmental pressure monitoring is of value in the unconscious patient, otherwise patients suspected of having compartment syndrome should be assessed for consideration of fasciotomy and decompression of all four compartments.

Open tibial fractures

There are published guidelines by the British Orthopaedic Association and British Association of Plastic Surgeons (1997) on the initial treatment of open tibial fractures to improve the prognosis for these patients. The wound is initially assessed, a swab taken for bacterial culture and a digital or Polaroid photograph taken of the wound (this allows for documentation of the initial injury and prevents constantly disturbing the wound to allow others to view it).

The wound is then dressed with an iodine-soaked dressing. Ideally, the most experienced clinician should assess the wound, taking into account Gustilo's criteria for descriptive purposes, thereafter with surgical colleagues.

Prophylactic broad-spectrum antibiotics are administered intravenously (usually 1.5g cefuroxime, with the addition of 500mg metronidazole and gentamicin, appropriately dosed, depending on the degree of wound contamination). The patient should also receive anti-tetanus medication as appropriate. The patient will require thorough surgical debridement and lavage of the wound to reduce the bone and soft tissue contamination and prevent infection from taking hold. If a plastic surgeon can be present for the initial debridement, further planning for soft tissue cover can be initiated. Evidence is lacking for immediate cover and traditionally should take place 3–5 days post-injury.

Conclusion

Tibial fractures are associated with high-energy trauma. The possible complications of this injury are numerous and frequent. Open fractures represent a significant proportion of these patients; morbidity associated with both open and closed injuries can be debilitating and commonly arise from injury to the soft tissues. The risk of chronic infection after open fractures of the tibia should be appreciated. Proper assessment and early involvement of appropriate expertise in the treatment of tibial fractures is the key to successful outcomes.

Key points

- Tibial fractures are common lower limb injuries.
- Careful evaluation is required to monitor for symptoms of compartment syndrome.
- Initial treatment requires fracture reduction and above-knee backslab application.
- Definitive treatment is dictated by fracture configuration and stability.
- Open injuries necessitate thorough surgical debridement and lavage before skeletal stabilisation.

References

British Orthopaedic Association and British Association of Plastic Surgeons (1997) *The Management of Open Tibial Fractures*. BOA/BAPS Working Party, London

Gustilo RB, Anderson JT (1976) Prevention of infection in the treatment of one thousand and twenty-five open fractures of long bones. *J Bone Joint Surg* **58-A**: 453–8

CHAPTER 23

Ankle fractures

Sam Oussedik

Anatomy and function

The ankle joint comprises three bones, the tibia, fibula and talus, together with the ligamentous structures that bind them together. Three groups of ligaments can be distinguished: the deltoid ligament medially, between tibia and talus; the lateral collateral ligaments laterally, comprising anterior talofibular, calcaneofibular and posterior talofibular ligaments; and the syndesmosis complex, comprising the interosseous membrane between tibia and fibula, anterior tibiofibular, posterior tibiofibular, inferior transverse and interosseous ligaments (*Figure 23.1*). Together, these structures allow movement of the talus within the mortise joint formed by tibia and fibula of 30° of dorsiflexion and 45° of plantar flexion.

Stability of the ankle joint, or its ability to maintain normal anatomical relationships between the bony structures through a range of motion, is conferred by both bony and ligamentous integrity. Accurately assessing fracture stability will therefore rely on identification of both bony and ligamentous injuries.

Two arteries cross the ankle joint to supply the foot, the anterior and posterior tibial arteries. Ensuring the presence of foot pulses is of paramount importance in assessing potential fracture dislocations of the ankle.

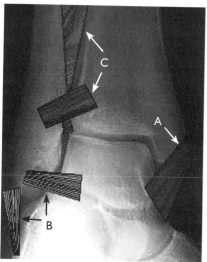

Figure 23.1. Schematic representation of ligaments of the ankle joint. The deltoid ligament (A), the lateral collateral ligaments (B). Anterior talofibular, calcaneofibular (shown) and posterior talofibular ligaments (not shown). The syndesmosis complex (C) (the interosseous membrane, anterior tibiofibular and interosseous ligaments (shown); the posterior tibiofibular and inferior transverse ligaments (not shown).

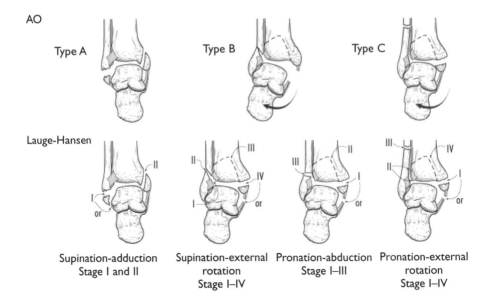

AO

Type A

Type B

Type C

Lauge-Hansen

Supination-adduction	Supination-external	Pronation-abduction	Pronation-external
Stage I and II	rotation	Stage I–III	rotation
	Stage I–IV		Stage I–IV

Figure 23.2. Ankle fracture classification – the relationship between the AO–Danis–Weber and Lauge-Hansen systems.

Mechanisms of injury

Ankle fractures are commonly the result of a combination of axial and rotational forces. The foot acts as a lever, such that forces transmitted through it to the ankle are multiplied, resulting in potential injury. The commonly used Lauge–Hansen classification (1950) classifies these injuries according to the presumed mechanism of injury, each mechanism leading to a predictable combination of radiographical findings (*Figure 23.2*).

Clinical presentation

Patients with ankle fractures present in varying degrees of distress, ranging from an antalgic gait through to the inability to weight bear associated with severe discomfort. Ankle examination should proceed along the traditional model of 'look, feel, move'. Inspection will reveal swelling (*Figure 23.3*). This may be localised to the affected malleolus or more diffuse. The integrity of the skin must be assessed, paying attention to any blistering or tenting. Any gross deformity noted at this stage, suggestive of ankle dislocation, should be dealt with by immediate reduction before radiographical assessment.

Palpation for point tenderness over medial, lateral and posterior malleoli should be carried out. The fifth metatarsal should also be palpated to rule out associated injury. The entire length of the fibula must also be examined, as

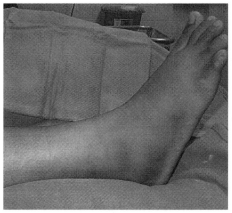

Figure 23.3. Appearance of an ankle fracture, with swelling and bruising over the lateral malleolus.

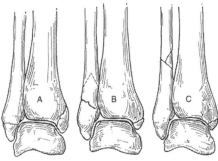

Figure 23.4. The AO–Danis–Weber classification of ankle fractures. Type A: a fibular fracture below the syndesmosis. Type B: a fibular fracture at the level of the syndesmosis. Type C: a fibular fracture above the syndesmosis.

associated fibula fractures can be found as high as the proximal tibiofibular articulation. Finally a neurovascular examination should be carried out, paying particular attention to the presence of dorsalis pedis and posterior tibial pulsations.

In assessing ankle injuries for the presence of a fracture, the Ottawa ankle rules should be applied (Stiell *et al*, 1992). These have been shown to be 100% sensitive and 40.1% specific in detecting malleolar fractures, and can be used to significantly reduce the number of radiographical studies requested. When applied to the ankle, these state that radiographs should only be requested for patients with pain in the malleolar zone and fulfilling either of the following criteria:

- Bony tenderness at the posterior edge of distal 6cm or tip of medial or lateral malleolus
- Inability to weight bear both immediately after injury and in the accident and emergency department by walking four steps.

For patients fulfilling the above criteria, mortise and lateral view radiographs should be requested.

Classification of injuries

Two classification systems are in common usage: the AO–Danis–Weber (Mueller *et al*, 1990) and the Lauge-Hansen (Lauge-Hansen, 1950). The former is the simpler of the two, classifying injuries according to the level of the fibular fracture alone: the more proximal the fracture, the greater the chance of associated instability (*Figure 23.4*).

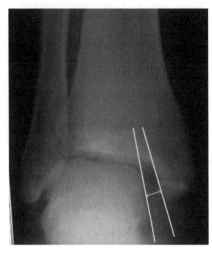

Figure 23.5. Lateral talar shift. The medial clear space has increased following a lateral malleolar fracture, indicating deltoid ligament injury and instability.

While this system does provide some information as to the nature of the injury, and thus aids communication between clinicians, it ignores the medial side.

The Lauge-Hansen (1950) classification is more comprehensive, but as a result is less easily applied. Injuries are classified according to the pattern of injury, which relates to a specific mechanism. These categories are the result of the author's cadaveric experiments. Each configuration is defined by two factors: the position of the foot (pronation or supination) and the force applied to the ankle (adduction, external rotation or abduction). In addition each configuration has a number of stages describing sequential injuries as force is applied:

- Supination-adduction – transverse lateral malleolar fracture below the tibial plafond and vertical shearing fracture of the medial malleolus.
- Supination-external rotation – anterior syndesmotic injury, oblique fibular fracture at the level of the plafond, medial malleolar fracture or deltoid avulsion, posterior syndesmotic injury and posterior malleolar fracture.
- Pronation-abduction – medial malleolar or deltoid avulsion, anterior syndesmotic injury, interosseous membrane tear, high fibular fracture.
- Pronation-external rotation – medial malleolar or deltoid injury, syndesmotic injury, bending fracture of fibula above syndesmosis.

In assessing any ankle fracture, the following points should be noted:

- Open or closed injury.
- Location of fracture(s): lateral malleolus (Weber A, B or C), medial malleolus or posterior malleolus.
- Displacement of fragments.
- Talar shift (*Figure 23.5*).

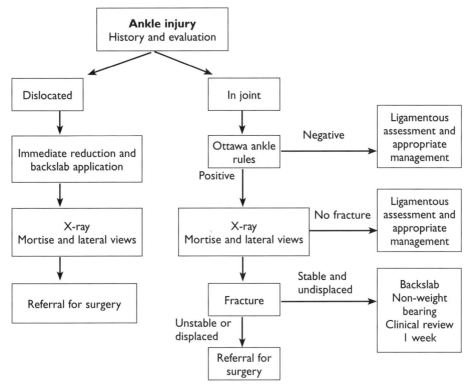

Figure 23.6. Summary of suggested management of ankle injuries.

These points, together with the overall clinical picture, will help to make a decision as to fracture stability and therefore the appropriate management regimen.

Management

As illustrated in *Figure 23.6*, initial management will depend on whether the ankle is in joint or not. A fracture-dislocation of the ankle requires emergency reduction and stabilisation in a backslab plaster before any radiographical assessment. Emergency reduction is necessary in order to minimise injury to the talus, remove excess pressure from the skin and ensure normal arterial supply to the foot. This can be carried out under sedation, ensuring adequate analgesics are also provided. However, if there is any doubt as to the integrity of the vascular supply to the foot then it may be necessary to relocate the ankle without sedation, although entonox should be provided.

The patient should be warned that he/she may feel a sharp increase in discomfort before relief. The deformity should be examined and an attempt made to reverse it. The heel is held in one hand while the other supports the

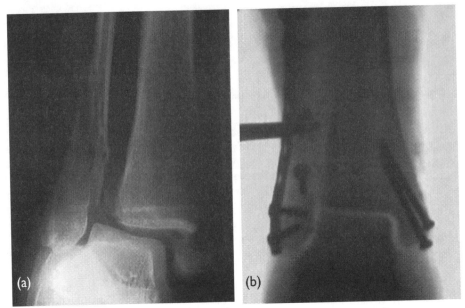

Figure 23.7. (a) A bi-malleolar displaced ankle fracture. (b) The same fracture following open reduction and internal fixation.

calf. Once normal ankle contours have been achieved, the ankle is supported in the reduced position while a plaster of Paris backslab is applied. At this stage radiographs can be requested. This should be followed by prompt orthopaedic referral for further management.

Ankle fractures which are not dislocated at presentation require assessment of stability to decide on appropriate management. Isolated undisplaced Weber A and B lateral malleolar fractures which do not show signs of instability, such as talar shift or evidence of deltoid ligament injury, can be managed by the application of a backslab and the provision of oral analgesics and crutches. Patients should be kept non-weight bearing for the initial post-injury period until fracture clinic review and advised to keep the ankle elevated as much as possible for the first week.

Displaced or unstable fractures require open reduction and internal fixation. Patients with injuries falling into this category should still receive adequate analgesia and the application of a backslab for comfort. Additionally, medial malleolar fractures are often treated operatively as there is a risk of non-union associated with non-operative management. Prompt orthopaedic review should be requested, as surgery can be delayed if too much swelling has accumulated making skin incisions difficult to close.

Operative management involves anatomical reduction of the fracture together with rigid fixation, usually with a combination of plates and screws (*Figures 23.7*).

Conclusions

Fracture-dislocations of the ankle require emergency reduction and immobilisation. Patients who present with ankle injuries which are not dislocated should be assessed by application of the Ottawa ankle rules. Those who go on to have a fracture diagnosed require assessment as to the stability of the injury. Classification aids this process, through the accurate application of either AO–Danis–Weber or Lauge-Hansen systems. Unstable and/or displaced fractures require operative management.

Key points

- Injuries to the ankle are among the most common encountered in the accident and emergency department.
- Fracture dislocations require prompt reduction.
- Accurate classification aids decision making when considering operative management.

References

Lauge-Hansen N (1950) Fractures of the ankle: II. Combined experimental-surgical and experimental roentgenologic investigations. *Arch Surg* **60**: 957–85

Mueller ME, Nazarian S, Koch P, Schatzker J (1990) *The Comprehensive Classification of Fractures of Long Bones*. Springer-Verlag, Berlin

Stiell IG, Greenberg GH, McNight RD, Nair RC, McDowell I, Worthington JR (1992) A study to develop clinical decision rules for the use of radiography in acute ankle injuries. *Arch Emerg Med* **21**: 384–90

Figure 23.3 is reproduced courtesy of www.emedx.com and *Figure 23.4* courtesy of http://www.orthoteers.co.uk

CHAPTER 24

Achilles tendon rupture

Rahul Patel and Fares Haddad

Introduction

The Achilles tendon, coined after the mythological Greek hero, is the largest and strongest tendon in the human body. The true prevalence of Achilles tendon rupture is unknown, although it occurs more commonly in men who are in their third to fifth decade of life and who participate in recreational activities. It is important to bear in mind the spectrum of Achilles tendon pathology (peritenonitis, tendinosis, and peritenonitis with tendinosis): the most common Achilles tendon injuries are Achilles tendinosis (formerly called Achilles tendonitis) and Achilles tendon rupture; the latter only will be discussed here.

Anatomy and function

The Achilles tendon (*Figure 24.1*) is the tendon that connects the calf muscle (gastrocnemius) to the heel bone (calcaneus). This is the tendon that is just below the skin at the back of the ankle.

When the gastrocnemius muscle contracts (shortens), the tendon which is attached from the muscle to the calcaneus, moves. As the muscle shortens, the tendon moves to point the foot downwards (plantarflexion). This is the action that allows a person to stand on his or her toes, to run, to jump, to walk normally, and to go up and down stairs. The Achilles tendon, the largest tendon in the body, is vulnerable to injury because of its limited blood supply and the combination of forces to which it is subjected. Aging and increased activity (particularly velocity

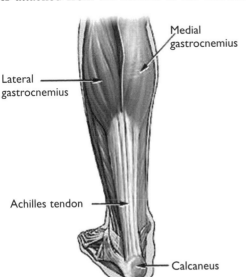

Lateral gastrocnemius

Medial gastrocnemius

Achilles tendon

Calcaneus

Figure 24.1. Anatomy of the Achilles tendon (posterior view).

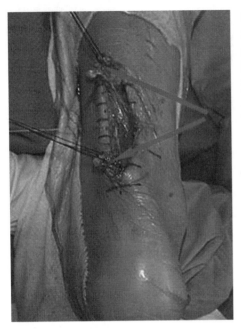

Figure 24.2 Ruptured ends of Achilles tendon.

sports) increase the chance of injury to the Achilles tendon. The blood supply to the tendon is provided by longitudinal arteries that run the length of the muscle complex. The area of the tendon with the poorest blood supply is approximately 2–6cm above the insertion into the calcaneus. The blood supply diminishes with age, predisposing this area of the tendon to chronic inflammation and possible rupture.

The Achilles tendon does not have a true synovial sheath but instead has a paratenon. The paratenon is a connective tissue sheath that surrounds the entire tendon and is able to stretch 2–3cm with movement, which allows maximal gliding action. The Achilles tendon has been shown to thicken in response to increased activity. The morphological changes such as decreased cell density, decreased collagen fibril density, and loss of fibre waviness that occur with aging predispose the tendon to injury.

The normal gait cycle requires extreme motion from within the ankle. With each step, the subtalar joint typically moves 30° (inverts 20°, everts 10°). This movement results in repetitive lengthening and shortening of the Achilles tendon complex. Running and jumping further increase the load on the Achilles tendon. Tendons that transmit large loads under these conditions are subject to injury. Extreme shear forces across the tendon complex are believed to cause prolonged loading of the tendon, resulting in microtrauma and inflammation, increasing vulnerability for consequent rupture.

Mechanism of injury

Ruptures of the Achilles tendon (*Figure 24.2*) most commonly occur spontaneously in healthy, young, active individuals who are aged 30–50 years and have no antecedent history of calf or heel pain. Unlike tears or ruptures at the musculotendinous junction of the Achilles tendon (tennis leg).

Poor conditioning, advanced age, and overexertion are risk factors for this injury. However, the common precipitating event is a sudden eccentric force applied to a dorsiflexed foot. Ruptures of the Achilles tendon also may occur as the result of direct trauma or as the end result following Achilles peritenonitis with or without tendinosis. Certain illnesses (such as arthritis and diabetes) and medications (such as corticosteroids and some antibiotics) can also increase the risk of rupture.

Injury often occurs during recreational sports that require bursts of jumping, pivoting, and running. A forceful push-off with the foot while the knee is straightened by the powerful thigh muscles is a common mechanism. One example might be starting a foot race or jumping.

A sudden trip or stumble, when the foot is thrust in front to break the fall, forcefully overstretching the tendon, is another mechanism associated with rupture as is a fall from a significant height.

Clinical picture and investigations

Delayed or missed diagnosis of Achilles tendon rupture is common, with 23% of patients initially being misdiagnosed (Inglis and Sculco, 1981). Therefore this diagnosis must always be born in mind and looked for when assessing Achilles pain or injury.

The diagnosis is made following an appropriate history and physical examination. The patient often presents with a sensation of a sudden snap in the back of the calf or heel that is associated with acute severe pain. This pain may be the result of an indirect injury (eccentric ankle contraction in a dorsiflexed foot) or a direct injury from blunt trauma to the tendon.

Antecedent pain in the back of the calf or heel may be an indication of prior tendon damage and vulnerability (eg. tendinitis, tendinosis, tenonitis).

The patient may have only minimal pain and may limp. Ankle weakness or apprehension manifests as the patient is unable to run, climb stairs, or stand on toes. The patient is unable to generate a strong posterior muscle contraction to plantar flex the ankle or foot.

Patients may have been told or may have thought the injury was a bad sprain because some active plantar flexion at the ankle may occur due to function of the intact posterior tibialis tendon, peroneal muscles, or flexor hallucis tendons; therefore, patients may present late.

Misdiagnosis or delayed treatment may result in a more difficult recovery period. Calf swelling may be evident.

For physical examination, the patient should lie prone on the examination table, with the knee flexed on the injured side. Palpation along the entire gastrocnemius-soleus musculotendinous unit to note tenderness, ecchymosis, swelling, and tendon defects should be performed. In patients with complete ruptures, a palpable gap along the Achilles tendon 2–6cm above its insertion may be noted. The Thompson test should be performed on all patients with suspected Achilles tendon injury. While the patient is prone and the affected

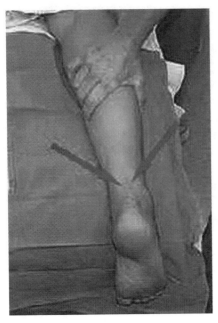

Figure 24.3. Thompson test.

leg is extended, the calf muscles are squeezed to indirectly plantar flex the foot. A positive Thompson test results if the foot does not plantar flex. A positive Thompson test helps confirm the diagnosis of a rupture (*Figure 24.3*).

Other tests are described and may aid diagnosis in equivocal cases, but are not performed routinely:

Hyperdorsiflexion sign: While the patient is prone and has both knees flexed to 90°, the ankles are maximally dorsiflexed passively and the injured side compared to the uninjured side.

O'Brien needle test: A small-gauge needle is inserted perpendicularly through the skin into the tendon substance, approximately 10cm proximal to the calcaneal insertion of the Achilles tendon. Motion of the hub of the needle in a direction opposite the tendon during passive ankle dorsiflexion and plantar flexion confirms an intact tendon distal to the needle level.

Radiographs are necessary to exclude avulsion type injury or any other concomitant foot or ankle fracture. X-rays of the ankle may show soft tissue swelling, increased ankle dorsiflexion, calcifications, a Haglund deformity, or bony metaplasia.

The diagnosis is mainly a clinical one but in equivocal cases other modalities of imaging may be helpful.

Ultrasound and magnetic resonance imaging (MRI) help confirm the diagnosis, but these studies are more helpful when partial tendon ruptures are suspected. Ultrasound and MRI are not routinely ordered for tendon ruptures.

Ultrasound is a relatively inexpensive, fast, repeatable, dynamic examination that helps determine tendon thickness and gap size. Ultrasound is operator-dependent and requires an experienced ultrasound technician and radiologist for reliable imaging.

MRI is more sensitive when trying to detect incomplete tendon ruptures (*Figure 24.4*), chronic degenerative changes, and fluid. In addition, MRI is able to discern peritenonitis, bursitis, tendon thickening, and rupture and can be used to monitor tendon healing. However, due to the high cost, limited clinical value, and inability to offer dynamic testing, MRI is not routinely indicated in patients with tendon ruptures.

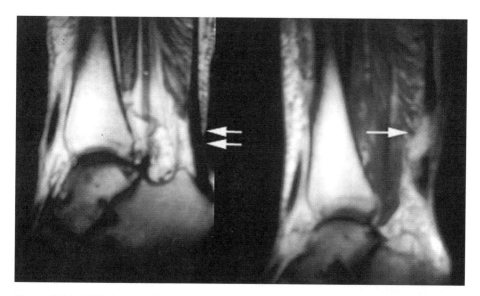

Figure 24.4. MRI showing Achilles tendon rupture..

Management

Initial

In the emergency department treatment for a rupture is simple. Even if a rupture is suspected but cannot be confirmed by other imaging, the injury should be treated as a rupture until confirmation can be obtained.

A plaster of Paris cast should be applied which holds the foot in maximal plantarflexion. This approximates the ruptured ends of the tendon and healing processes can begin with the tendon anatomically reduced. This may be crucial if conservative treatment (sequential casting) is chosen. If there is calf swelling or vulnerable skin around the ankle an anterior plaster slab may be preferred.

The patient is advised to be strictly non-weight bearing and given crutches. Elevation and anti-inflammatory medication form the remainder of acute treatment.

Referral to an orthopaedic surgeon is mandatory so that definitive treatment may be discussed and effected. Although there is no strong evidence to support that immediate surgical repair is superior to early repair, discussion with the surgeon as soon as possible is suggested.

Definitive

Treatment of Achilles tendon rupture is controversial. The principal treatment is surgery plus immobilisation, or immobilisation alone (conservative). The

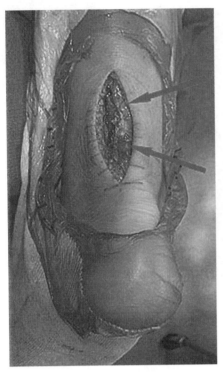

Figure 24.5. Repaired Achilles tendon.

goal of the orthopaedic surgeon is to restore tendon continuity and length to allow patients to regain their functional and desired activity level.

Acute ruptures, large partial ruptures, and re-ruptures are indications for surgical repair. On the other hand, patients who are more elderly and/or more inactive and those who have systemic illnesses or poor skin integrity are not optimal candidates for operative treatment and are better served with non-operative treatment. In general, we recommend operative intervention for younger, healthier, more active individuals who desire a reliable treatment method. Individuals participating in semi-professional or professional sports are strongly encouraged to have surgery to decrease the chance of re-rupture and to optimise outcome in terms of push-off strength and successful return to activity.

Numerous operative procedures are available to repair the Achilles tendon. Open and closed (percutaneous) procedures are described (*Figure 24.5*). These procedures usually involve primary end-to-end tendon repair with or without fascial or tendon reinforcement.

Advantages of operative treatment include a lower re-rupture rate, a higher percentage of patients to return to sports, and a greater return of strength, endurance, and power (Cetti *et al*, 1993).

Disadvantages of operative treatment include hospitalisation, high operative costs, wound complications (eg. infection, skin slough, and sinus formation), adhesions, and possible sural nerve injury (especially through a lateral longitudinal approach).

Both methods of treatment require immobilisation (non-weight bearing) for a lengthy period. For conservative treatment, the patient is fully plantar flexed for approximately 4 weeks and then sequentially casted with increasing dorsiflexion until a neutral position is reached, over 6 weeks.

Post-surgical patients may require a shorter period fully plantar flexed (2–3 weeks) and are similarly sequentially casted until a neutral position is reached over approximately 6 weeks. However, newer surgical rehabilitation techniques obviate the need for plaster of Paris after 2–4 weeks and include the use thereafter of specialised removable boots with built up heels (heel wedges) which are sequentially reduced, or specialised ankle braces which limit range of motion initially and then gradually increase it. Reliable evidence for these newer modalities of rehabilitation is emerging.

Physiotherapy forms the mainstay of treatment thereafter where gait, strength, stamina and propioception are addressed.

Conclusion

Achilles tendon rupture is a relatively common injury sustained during sporting activity, in the main, by non-professional athletes. The history and examination usually lead to the diagnosis but investigations such as ultrasound or MRI can confirm rupture. Treatment can be non-operative or operative each with varying risks, but the latter is preferred in younger, more active patients.

Key points

- The Achilles tendon, the largest tendon in the body, is vulnerable to injury because of its limited blood supply and the combination of forces to which it is subjected.
- Aging and increased activity (particularly velocity sports) increase the chance of injury to the Achilles tendon.
- Extreme shear forces across the tendon complex are believed to cause prolonged loading of the tendon, resulting in microtrauma and inflammation, increasing vulnerability for consequent rupture.
- Ruptures of the Achilles tendon most commonly occur spontaneously in healthy, young, active individuals who are aged 30–50 years and have no antecedent history of calf or heel pain.
- Delayed or missed diagnosis of Achilles tendon rupture is common.
- A positive Thompson test results if the foot does not plantar flex. A positive Thompson test helps confirm the diagnosis of a rupture.
- Ultrasound and MRI are not routinely ordered for tendon ruptures.
- Even if a rupture is suspected but cannot be confirmed by other imaging, the injury should be treated as a rupture until confirmation can be obtained.
- A plaster of Paris cast should be applied which holds the foot in maximal plantarflexion.
- The principal treatment is surgery plus immobilisation, or immobilisation alone (conservative).

References

Cetti R, Christensen SE, Ejsted R, Jensen NM, Jorgensen U (1993) Operative versus nonoperative treatment of Achilles tendon rupture. A prospective randomized study and review of the literature. *Am J Sports Med* **21(6)**: 791–9

Inglis AE, Sculco TP (1981) Surgical repair of ruptures of the tendo-achilles. *Clin Orthop Relat Res* **156**: 160–9

CHAPTER 25

Hind foot fractures of the calcaneus and talus

Aklbar De Medici, Sam Oussedik and Fares Haddad

Introduction

The foot has two vital functions, first to support the body while standing or walking and second to act as a lever in propelling the body forward. Hence any damage to the structures that make up the foot will have a significant impact on its function. Fractures of the hind foot are not uncommon and make up 2% of all fractures seen in adults. They are frequently missed, especially osteochondral fractures and fractures of the lateral and posterior processes of the talus which are radiographically difficult to detect. Controversies remain over the ideal management of these fractures and no one surgical strategy has eliminated the often significant long-term disability associated with these injuries. These difficulties make hind foot fractures an area of potential disaster, both for the patient and doctor.

Anatomy and function of the hind foot

The importance of fractures of the hind foot become apparent once the anatomy is appreciated (*Figure 25.1*). The principal bones of the hind foot are the talus and calcaneus. These two bones make up the central components in the ankle, subtalar and midtarsal joints. Any of these joints may be involved in the injury.

Ankle joint

The ankle joint is made up of the tibia, fibula and talus, and is a synovial hinge joint. The articular surfaces are enclosed by the joint capsule, reinforced by collateral ligaments. This allows dorsiflexion and plantarflexion movements only.

Subtalar joint

The subtalar joint is made up of:

- The talocalcaneal joint – the articulation of the upper surface of the calcaneus with the lower surface of the talus (synovial plane joint).

Calcaneus
Talus
Sustentaculum tali
Facet for medial malleolus

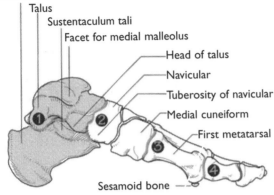

Head of talus
Navicular
Tuberosity of navicular
Medial cuneiform
First metatarsal

Sesamoid bone

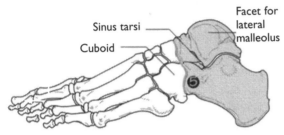

Sinus tarsi
Cuboid

Facet for lateral malleolus

Figure 25.1 Medial and lateral images of the bones of the foot. The main joints are: 1: subtalar; 2: midtarsal (talonavicular); 3: Tarsometatarsal; 4: Metatarsophalangeal; 5: Midtarsal (calcaneocuboid). The region of the hind foot is shaded.

- The talocalcaneonavicular joint – the articulation between the head of talus and the sustentaculum tali (synovial ball and socket joint).

This joint allows eversion and inversion movements.

Midtarsal joint

The midtarsal joint is made up of:

- The calcaneocuboid joint – the articulation of the anterior surface of the calcaneus and the posterior surface of the cuboid (synovial plane joint).
- The talonavicular component of the talocalcaneonavicular joint.

This joint assists with eversion and inversion movements.

Hind foot fractures

Calcaneal fractures

The os calcis is the most frequently fractured tarsal bone (more than 60% of tarsal fractures). Calcaneal fractures are most commonly seen in young men. They are often bilateral (~10%) (Lance *et al*, 1964) owing to the mechanism of injury which is usually a high energy axial force (Carr, 1993) directed through the laterally situated plantar tuberosity of the calcaneum. Hence there are often other associated fractures, eg. compression fractures of the lumbar spine (~10%) and other lower limb fractures (~26%) (Cave, 1963). Other recognised mechanisms of injury include motor vehicle collisions, blunt-force injury causing extra-articular fractures of the calcaneal body and plantar tuberosity, abrupt contraction of the Achilles tendon causing avulsion injuries, and stress fractures in athletes. Open fractures are rare (<2%).

Talar fractures

The rate of reported fracture of the talus is about 2% of all foot fractures, making it rare. However, the implications of this fracture are huge as the talus is one of the most important bones in the functioning of the foot. It also has a rather tenuous blood supply, making it vulnerable to injury or interruption, and three-fifths is covered by articular cartilage, hence avascular necrosis and arthritis are common complications. It is therefore important to recognise these injuries and treat them appropriately to avoid these complications. The usual mechanism of injury is sudden hyperextension of the foot. They often occur in young athletes, but should be suspected at any age and are usually the result of a motor vehicle accident or fall from height.

Documentation of the history should include:

- *Mechanism of injury*. This will focus the attention to the correct area, highlight other potential injuries and indicate severity.
- *Age*. This will affect the type of injury, outcome and treatment.
- *Occupation*. As hind foot fractures have significant morbidity, those patients whose occupation involves walking and/or in which balance is important should be forewarned of possible long-term difficulties.
- *Smoking and comorbidity*. These will affect surgical management.

Examination of the hind foot

The basic rules of look, feel and move still apply:

- *Look*: Swelling, widening of heel, bruising often medially (*Figure 25.2*).
- *Feel*: Local tenderness.
- *Move*: Unable to weight bear.

Talar fractures are more difficult to diagnose clinically, but the history is key and the patient cannot usually weight bear comfortably or at all. Calcaneal fractures are usually more dramatic.

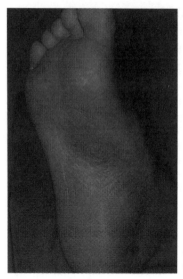

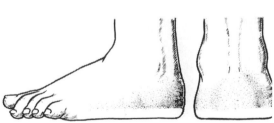

Figure 25.2. Bruising and swelling seen with calcaneal fractures.

Investigations

Once a hind foot fracture is suspected all patients should have their foot elevated and supported, and analgesia should be given until the diagnosis is proven or excluded.

The first-line investigation is plain film radiography. This should include the following views:

- Ankle/hind foot anteroposterior and lateral.
- Axial projection (to visualise the heel).
- If a talar fracture is suspected films may be taken in plantar and dorsiflexion to aid the diagnosis.

Bohler's angle (Bohler, 1931) (*Figure 25.3*) is a line drawn along the superior border of the posterior part of calcaneal body and one drawn from the anterior articular process of the calcaneum through the posterior articular facet of the subtalar joint. If Bohler's angle is 35°–40° the calcaneus is normal, if it is <40° (often 0°) the calcaneus is fractured. Having confirmed the diagnosis through plain film radiography, computed tomography may be of great use in planning possible surgery.

Fracture classification

For the purposes of accident and emergency the following rule of thumb can be applied to hind foot fractures.

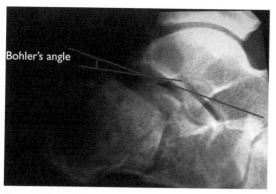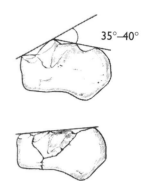

Figure 25.3. Measurement of Bohler's angle.

- Is there a fracture – yes/no?
- If so, which bone – calcaneum or talus?
- If talus, refer as there is a high likelihood of long-term complication.
- If the calcaneum – is it intra- or extra-articular?
- If intra-articular (70%) this needs referral as there is a high rate of complications.
- Extra-articular fractures are mostly treated conservatively unless they are displaced, in which case advice should be sought.

Talar fractures

Talar fractures fall into three groups:

- Fracture of the body.
- Fracture through the neck (50%): types I–IV (Hawkins classification) (*Table 25.1*).
- Osteochondral fractures.

Unfortunately all these fractures carry a high risk of long-term complications such as avascular necrosis or arthritis, therefore all need orthopaedic review. Many will be treated conservatively, some by open reduction and internal fixation, but most will be non-weight bearing for several weeks.

Calcaneal fractures

The pattern of injury seen will determine treatment and falls into seven main categories which are summarised in *Table 25.2*. These can be extra- or intra-articular. Extra-articular fractures tend naturally to have a better prognosis.

Table 25.1. Hawkins classification of talar neck fractures

Radiographic findings	Risk of AVN
Type I Non-displaced fracture line	0–13%
Type II Displaced fracture, plus subluxation or dislocation of subtalar joint	20–50%
Type III Displaced fracture, dislocation subtalar and tibiotalar joints	69–100%
Type IV Displaced fracture and disruption of talonavicular joint	High

AVN = avascular necrosis

More than one injury usually always warrants referral, and soft tissue or neurovascular injuries must not be overlooked.

Many systems have been used to describe these fractures including the Sanders classification and the Essex-Lopresti (1993) system.

Long-term outcome

Most studies have found a very poor long-term outcome in the more serious fractures of the hind foot (Hildebrand *et al*, 1996; Loucks and Buckley, 1999). There is not yet an answer as to which treatment offers the best outcome as both conservative and surgical options have been shown to have beneficial results (Buckley *et al*, 2002). Each case has to be taken on its own merit and if in doubt senior review should be sought as mistakes can be costly.

Key points

- Fractures of the hind foot account for around 2% of those seen in adults.
- The hind foot comprises a number of joints the integrity of which is vital for pain-free walking.
- Accurate diagnosis and prompt management will help to achieve an optimal outcome.

References

Bohler L (1931) Diagnosis, pathology, and treatment of fractures of the os calcis. *J Bone Joint Surg* **13**: 75–89

Buckley R, Tough S, McCormack R, Pate G, Leighton R, Petrie D, Galpin R (2002) Operative

Table 25.2. The common classification of calcaneal fractures, their treatment, outcomes and which to refer

Fracture type	Early treatment	Late treatment	Outcome
Vertical fracture of tuberosity*	Tight bandage, elevation	Loose bandage and crutches	Good
Horizontal fracture Non-avulsion	Manipulation	Below knee plaster and crutches (5 weeks)	Healing by 5 weeks
Avulsion†	Elevation – refer for surgery	Open reduction and internal fixation	Healing by 8 weeks
Fractures of the sustentaculum tali*	Crepe bandage Below-knee cast	NWB for 6 weeks Crutches and/or walking heel	Healing by 6–8 weeks
Anterior calcaneal fractures‡	Treat as for fracture of sustentaculum tali unless calcaneal shortening or midtarsal instability – refer		Healing by 6–8 weeks
Fracture of the body no displacement‡	Pressure bandaging, bedrest and elevation. Refer for review (may need pinning)	Crutches and touch weight bearing	Good, may have residual heel pain
Fractures of the body with displacement and subtalar involvement†	Conservative vs surgery? All need referral		Poor
Central crushing fractures†	Need referral	Often long-term complications need follow up	Poor

*Relatively stable or safe fracture which can be reliably treated conservatively; †those that need inpatient management or specialist review and are usually intra-articular; ‡those fractures that must be handled carefully and should be reviewed by an orthopaedic specialist on admission. NWB = non weight-bearing

compared with nonoperative treatment of displaced intra-articular calcaneal fractures: a prospective, randomized, controlled multicenter trial. *J Bone Joint Surg Am* **84-A(10)**: 1733–44

Carr JB (1993) Mechanisms and pathoanatomy of the intraarticular calcaneal fracture. *Clin Orthop* **290**: 36–40

Cave EF (1963) Fracture of the os calcis – the problem in general. *Clin Orthop* **30**: 64–6

Essex-Lopresti P (1993) The mechanism, reduction technique, and results in fractures of the os calcis, 1951–52. *Clin Orthop* **290**: 3–16

Hildebrand KA, Buckley RE, Mohtadi NGH, Faris P (1996) Functional outcome measures after displaced intra-articular calcaneal fractures. *J Bone Joint Surg (Br)* **78B**: 119–23

Lance EM, Carey EJ Jr, Wade PA (1964) Fractures of the os calcis: a follow up study. *J Trauma* **4**: 15–56

Loucks C, Buckley R (1999) Bohler's angle: correlation with outcome in displaced intra-articular calcaneal fractures. *J Ortho Trauma* **13(8)**: 554–8

Further reading

Barei DP, Bellabarba C, Sangeorzan BJ, Benirschke SK (2002) Fractures of the calcaneus. *Orthop Clin North Am* **33(1)**: 263–85

Bucholz RW (2005) (1996) *Rockwood and Green's Fractures in Adults*. Volume 2. Lippincott Williams and Wilkins, Philadelphia

Crosby LA, Kamins P (1991) The history of the calcaneal fracture. *Orthop Rev* **20**: 501–9

McRae R (2003) *Pocketbook of Orthopaedics and Fractures*. Churchill Livingstone, London

CHAPTER 26

Metatarsal fractures

Rahul Patel and Fares Haddad

Introduction

The forefoot serves two purposes during gait. First, as a unit, it provides a broad plantar surface for load sharing. The two sesamoids and four lesser metatarsal heads share an equal amount of the load in normal gait. Second, the forefoot is mobile in the sagittal plane, thus enabling the forefoot to change the position of the individual metatarsal heads to accommodate uneven ground.

Metatarsal fractures usually result from a direct blow of a heavy object dropped onto the forefoot. However indirect forces, particularly twisting the body with the toes fixed, apply torque to the foot, producing fractures of the metatarsal shafts. Fractures particular to individual metatarsals will be discussed briefly as will stress fractures.

Anatomy and function

The human foot combines mechanical complexity and structural strength.

Structurally, the foot has three main parts: the forefoot, the midfoot, and the hindfoot. The forefoot is composed of the five toes (called phalanges) and their connecting long bones (metatarsals).

The foot has two important functions: weight bearing and propulsion. These functions require a high degree of stability. In addition, the foot must be flexible, so it can adapt to uneven surfaces. The multiple bones and joints of the foot give it flexibility, but these multiple bones must form an arch to support any weight.

The foot has three arches. The medial longitudinal arch is the highest and most important of the three arches. It is composed of the calcaneus, talus, navicular, cuneiforms, and the first three metatarsals. The lateral longitudinal arch is lower and flatter than the medial arch. It is composed of the calcaneus, cuboid, and the fourth and fifth metatarsals. The transverse arch is composed of the cuneiforms, the cuboid, and the five metatarsal bases (trapezoid in cross-section). The second metatarsal base is regarded as the keystone of the arch and most important. The second tarsometatarsal joint is slightly recessed into the midfoot.

The arches of the foot are maintained not only by the shapes of the bones

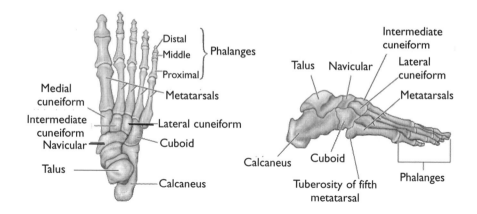

Figure 26.1. Top and lateral view of bones of the foot.

but also by ligaments. The lateral four metatarsals are connected to each other by strong intermetatarsal ligaments but are conspicuously absent between the first and second metatarsals. Instead, the base of the second metatarsal is joined to the first tarsometatarsal joint by the medial interosseous ligament, or Lisfranc's ligament, connecting the plantar aspect of the second metatarsal base to the medial cuneiform. This represents the largest ligament in Lisfranc's joint complex and is responsible for the second metatarsal base avulsion often seen with Lisfranc's injuries. In addition, muscles and tendons play an important role in supporting the arches.

The phalanges are connected to the metatarsals by five metatarsal phalangeal joints at the ball of the foot. The forefoot bears half the body's weight and balances pressure on the ball of the foot (*Figure 26.1*).

The first metatarsal bone bears the most weight and plays the most important role in propulsion. It is the shortest and thickest. It also provides attachment for several tendons. The second and third metatarsals are relatively fixed in position within the foot; the first, fourth, and fifth are relatively mobile. More stress is placed on the second and third metatarsals when ambulating, so these are at increased risk for stress fracture. The fifth metatarsal, which is approximately 1.5cm from the proximal pole of the bone, bears greater stress in those who over supinate when they walk or run. The fifth metatarsal also has a diminished blood supply and thus, decreased ability to heal.

Radiological anatomy

On the anteroposterior view, the lateral border of the first metatarsal should be aligned with the lateral border of the medial cuneiform. The medial border of the second metatarsal should be aligned with the medial border of the intermediate cuneiform bone.

On the oblique view, the medial and lateral border of the third metatarsal should be aligned with the medial and lateral borders of lateral cuneiform bone. The medial border of the fourth metatarsal should be aligned with the medial border of the cuboid bone. The fourth and fifth metatarsals are aligned with the cuboid bone, but the lateral part of the fifth metatarsal can project beyond the margin of the cuboid bone, up to 3mm.

The distance between the base of the first and second metatarsals and the medial and intermediate cuneiform is more than the distance between other corresponding joints.

If a lateral image is obtained a line through the long axis of talus bone and the long axis of first metatarsal bone should be straight if there is no dislocation.

Mechanisms of injury

Metatarsal fractures are usually caused by the blow of a heavy object dropped onto the forefoot or by a twisting injury. Fractures of the shaft can be caused by twisting of the body with the toes fixed, applying torque to the foot.

Avulsion (pull-off) fractures occur particularly at the base of the fifth metatarsal. A Jones fracture (base of fifth metatarsal) is caused by inversion of foot, which produces tension on the peroneus brevis tendon and on the lateral cord of the plantar aponeurosis. In this type of fracture, significant displacement is absent. This type of fracture is more prone to nonunion.

Distal fractures, also called dancer's fractures, are caused by a rotational force caused by axial loading with the foot in a plantar flexed position.

The Lisfranc joints are the tarsometatarsal joints. A Lisfranc fracture dislocation is caused by falling from a height, falling down stairs, or stepping off a curb.

Mechanisms of injury are (1) rotation around a fixed forefoot (eg. falling from horse with the foot caught in the stirrup, the origin of the eponym) or (2) longitudinal compression of the foot. In this second mechanism, the metatarsal head is fixed, with the weight of the body on the hindfoot against the base of metatarsals along with rotation; these forces result in a distal dorsal dislocation of the metatarsal.

Stress fractures are common in the second and third metatarsal necks and at the proximal portion of the shaft of the fifth metatarsal. Athletes and soldiers seem to be more prone to this type of injury. Patients usually report increased intensity or duration of exercise regimen. Dull pain occurs initially only with exercise, progressing to pain at rest. The pain starts as diffuse, then localises to the site of the fracture.

A stress fracture is not the result of a single occurrence, but rather an ongoing process. They are rare before adolescence as is bilateral presentation. In sedentary individuals, the cause is usually related to unaccustomed activity.

Mechanisms may involve repetitive stress, usually as a result of frequent impact weight-bearing exercise eventually yielding to a fracture due to continued loading. Biomechanical abnormalities, such as excessive pronation, hypersupination, lower extremity malalignment, external or internal femoral rotation and limb length discrepancy can all lead to an alteration in normal gait, which can then lead to stress fractures.

Insufficiency fractures are due to normal stress on a weakened bone. This injury is seen in people with osteoporosis, and commonly affects postmenopausal women.

Clinical picture and investigations

The cardinal signs and symptoms are pain, deformity, crepitus, swelling, bruising and increased pain on weight bearing. In a fracture of the fifth metatarsal, pain and tenderness are present at the base of the fifth metatarsal, along with swelling, ecchymosis, and difficulty in weight bearing. This fracture is sometime hard to differentiate from an ankle injury because the swelling can be near the region of the lateral malleolus. The head of the second metatarsal head is most commonly affected, although other bones can be involved as well.

Proper history taking in patients with symptoms and suggestive mechanisms of injury is essential.

Radiography is the first and often the only investigation required for the diagnosis of fractures. Radiographs can be used diagnose all acute fractures, dislocations, and established stress fractures. Anteroposterior (AP), lateral and 30° oblique radiographs should be requested.

Bone scanning is more sensitive than plain radiography and indicated when a stress or acute fracture is suspected and radiographs are negative. Bone scanning is not a specific investigation.

Although magnetic resonance imaging (MRI) is more sensitive than radiography and bone scanning, it is used only for the assessment of soft tissue structures and ligamentous injuries. MRI is the most sensitive technique for imaging stress fractures of the foot and can depict bone marrow oedema even before increased uptake is seen on bone scans.

Computed tomography (CT) scanning is useful for finding avulsion fractures and comminuted fractures to assess for intra-articular extension.

Small avulsions can be missed on radiographs. In the early stages of stress fracture, radiographs can be normal, or they may show only subtle periosteal reaction, which can be easily missed. Radiography cannot be used to assess soft-tissue and ligamentous disruption.

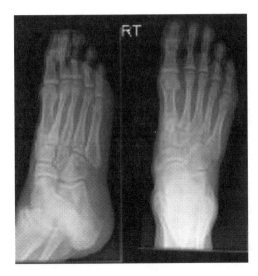

Figure 26.2. Spiral fracture of distal shaft of fifth metatarsal.

Although CT and MRI are more sensitive than radiography, they are not cost-effective and not indicated for the diagnosis of fractures. Bone scanning is sensitive but it can still miss some stress fractures in the early stages.

Classification systems

Many classifications apply to fracture of the fifth metatarsal.

A simple classification for fractures of the proximal end of the fifth metatarsal divides them into:

- Fractures of the tuberosity.
- Fractures of the proximal metatarsal within 1.5cm of the tuberosity.

Acute fractures, Jones fractures, and stress fractures can be described as early, delayed union, or nonunion fractures.

The Stewart classification (1960) of fifth metatarsal fractures is:

- Type I: extra-articular fracture between the metatarsal base and diaphysis.
- Type II: intra-articular fracture of the metatarsal base.
- Type III: avulsion fracture of the base.
- Type IV: comminuted fracture with intra-articular extension.
- Type V: partial avulsion of the metatarsal base with or without a fracture.

The zonal classification reported by Dameron (1975), and Lawrence and Botte (1993) categorises metatarsal fractures by the region affected: zone 1 corresponds to the tuberosity, zone 2 corresponds to Jones fractures and zone 3 is the diaphysis (*Figure 26.2*).

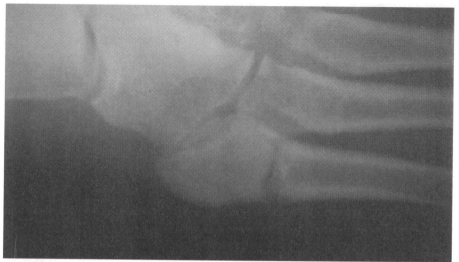

Figure 26.3. Jones fracture.

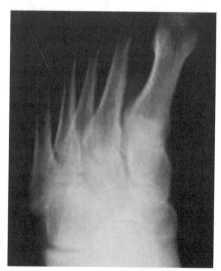

Figure 26.4. Fracture of proximal shaft of first metatarsal.

Common fractures

Fractures can affect any metatarsal, but the fifth metatarsal is most commonly affected. The fracture can be transverse, oblique or comminuted. Longitudinal linear fractures are extremely rare.

The two most common fractures in the fifth metatarsal are a fracture at the tip of the tuberosity and a transverse fracture 1.5–2cm from the tuberosity; the latter is called a Jones fracture (*Figure 26.3*).

The head of the first metatarsal is thought to bear one third of body weight. Three types of fracture predominate: avulsion, proximal shaft (*Figure 26.4*) and mid-shaft. Shorter and wider than the other metatarsals, it also has a lack of interconnecting ligaments between itself and the second metatarsal. This allows for independent motion.

Fractures of the middle metatarsals can be isolated or multiple (*Figures 26.5* and *26.6*). Oblique and transverse diaphyseal fractures predominate. With regard to treatment, emphasis, as with the first metatarsal, is on the resulting position of the metatarsal head.

Two types of Lisfranc dislocation have been described: homolateral

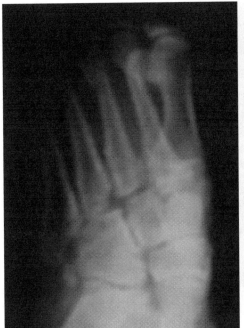

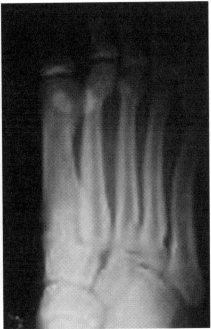

Figure 26.5. Fracture of distal shaft of third metatarsal.

Figure 26.6 Fractures of second and third metatarsal heads (oblique view).

and divergent (Quenu and Kuss, 1909). In the homolateral type, all of the metatarsals are dislocated to one side. Usually, the second to fifth metatarsals are dislocated, but occasionally, all of the metatarsals are affected.

Lisfranc dislocations are associated with fractures of the base of the second metatarsal, fractures of the cuboid bone, fractures of the shaft of the other metatarsal bones, dislocations of the middle and medial cuneonavicular joints, and fractures of the navicular bone. The base of the second metatarsal is relatively fixed compared with the other metatarsal bones. Therefore, it is involved in both types.

This dislocation is overlooked in as many as 20% of cases if the alignment is not carefully evaluated. There is a consistent relationship between the medial border of the second and fourth metatarsals and the medial edge of their corresponding cuneiform bones.

Lisfranc dislocations (*Figure 26.7* and *26.8*) should be suspected if a gap of more than 5mm is present between the bases of first and second metatarsals or between the medial and middle cuneiforms.

The radiographic findings of a stress fracture depend on the bone involved and the stage of disease. Radiographs are normal in the early stages of the disease, and stress fractures appear as well-defined linear lucency or fluffy

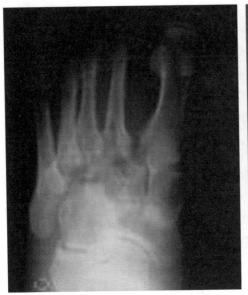

Figure 26.7. Lisfranc fracture-dislocation:
a fracture of the base of the second
metatarsal and a lateral dislocation of the
second metatarsal.

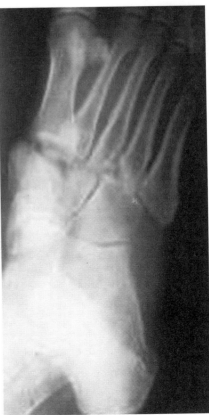

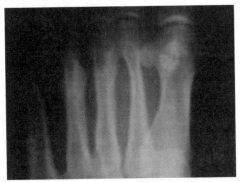

Figure 26.8. (above) Lisfranc
dislocation with a fracture of the base
of the third and fourth metatarsals.
Figure 26.9. (left) Stress fracture
with extensive periosteal reaction on
either side of the third and fourth
metatarsals.

periosteal reactions by 7–10 days. The periosteal reaction is variable and is occasionally florid (*Figure 26.9*).

The head of the second metatarsal, and occasionally the third metatarsal, are commonly affected. The first metatarsal is injured in only 10% of metatarsal stress fractures and involves a different kind of reaction (the endosteal variety), with linear sclerosis. Periosteal reaction is not common in this type of injury.

The base of the second metatarsals can be affected in ballet dancers. The proximal aspect of the shaft of the fourth and fifth metatarsals is affected, and the pattern is that of a linear lucency, which is slow to heal. Fractures in the sesamoid bones are also seen in ballet dancers.

Management

Initial and definitive

Base of fifth metatarsal fractures and Jones fractures can mostly be treated in non-weight bearing plaster of Paris casts for 6–8 weeks. However, it is advisable to arrange orthopaedic follow-up in all cases as some can progress to delayed or non-union and if significant displacement exists, should be considered for internal fixation. If symptoms are slight, a crepe bandage or similar support for 2–3 weeks is indicated. All athletes should be considered for internal fixation to facilitate early return to sport and minimise non-union rates.

Shaft fractures of the metatarsals should be assessed as any other fracture in terms of displacement and angulation. There are no fixed criteria for acceptable or unacceptable position of the head, but problems of transfer metatarsalgia and shoe wear are common if there are significant changes in the normal position of the head. Normally 10° of deviation in the dorsal/plantar plane or 3–4mm of translation in any plane requires active correction; manipulation or gravitational traction. An Aircast boot or a below knee plaster of Paris with weight bearing as tolerated, are the mainstay of conservative closed treatment thereafter.

Multiple adjacent fractures with significant soft tissue injury or fractures significantly displaced and angulated resistant to manipulation, require open reduction and fixation with K-wires. A plate may be used if the soft tissues are intact. Traction remains an option if control is difficult to achieve or the fracture extends into the head and metatarsophalangeal joint.

Conservative treatment or to hold position after fixation, is a short leg plaster of Paris cast for 4–6 weeks. This may be removable after the first two weeks. Position of the foot is as above. Weight bearing is encouraged on the heel, as tolerated.

All suspected Lisfranc injuries should be referred to the orthopaedic team immediately for assessment as the mainstay of treatment is open reduction and internal fixation. Closed reduction and percutaneous pinning may be attempted. Prognosis of Lisfranc injuries without fracture is poor due to late midfoot collapse.

Treatment of stress fractures depends on the time the diagnosis was made. In cases of fresh injury, rest, ice, elevation and compression (RICE) are very helpful as well as anti-inflammatory medication. An Aircast boot may be used if weight bearing is to be allowed, but an elastic bandage and non-weight bearing status is adequate. Both types of immobilisation, total rest and refrainment from exercise/sport for 4–8 weeks is necessary. Metaphyseal fractures heal quicker than articular or cortical ones.

Heat and fluido-therapy are helpful in increasing blood flow to the area, which can help to accelerate bone healing. The patient can begin rehabilitation when pain free, but not necessarily return to sporting activity. The patient must have full range of motion in the joints in the injured extremity, have redeveloped the flexibility of the muscles of that limb and developed strength, endurance, proprioception, agility and cardiovascular reserve before returning to full competition. A good training programme, the use of proper footwear, impact surfaces and orthoses can be important preventative measures to take in the recurrence of stress fractures. In the athlete, the stress fracture is the epitome of an overuse injury and, as such, signals the need to investigate training habits, equipment and athletic techniques.

Conclusion

Forefoot injuries are commonplace and thus an understanding of the spectrum of injury is important. The history and mechanism of injury usually make diagnosis straightforward aided by the correct investigatory modalities. The majority of forefoot fractures can be treated conservatively, but certainly the swelling associated with higher energy injuries may cause a compartment syndrome of the foot and should be examined and continually assessed for. Appropriate rehabilitation is paramount in the successful treatment of these injuries and thus physiotherapists and perhaps orthotists, play important roles in their management.

References

Dameron TB Jr (1975) Fractures and anatomical variations of the proximal portion of the fifth metatarsal. *J Bone Joint Surg Am* **57(6)**: 788–92

Lawrence SJ, Botte MJ (1993) Jones' fractures and related fractures of the proximal fifth metatarsal. *Foot Ankle* **14(6)**: 358–65

Quenu E, Kuss G (1909) Etude sur les luxations du metatose. *Rev Chir* **39**: 231–6

Stewart IM (1960) Jones's fracture: fracture of base of fifth metatarsal. *Clin Orthop Relat Res* **16**:190–8

Key points

- Structurally, the foot has three main parts: the forefoot, the midfoot, and the hindfoot.
- The foot has three arches: the medial longitudinal arch, the lateral longitudinal arch and the transverse arch. The arches of the foot are maintained by the shapes of the bones as well as by ligaments and muscles.
- The first metatarsal bone bears the most weight and plays the most important role in propulsion.
- More stress is placed on the second and third metatarsals when ambulating, so these are at increased risk for stress fracture.
- Radiological appearances of normal anatomy must be borne in mind when assessing X-rays.
- Metatarsal fractures are usually caused by the blow of a heavy object dropped onto the forefoot or by a twisting injury.
- Avulsion (pull-off) fractures occur particularly at the base of the fifth metatarsal.
- Lisfranc injuries are often missed. Expert opinion should be sought if there is any doubt as improper management leads to significant morbidity.
- Stress fractures are common in the second and third metatarsal necks and at the proximal portion of the shaft of the fifth metatarsal. Mechanisms may involve repetitive stress, usually as a result of frequent impact weight-bearing exercise eventually yielding to a fracture due to continued loading.
- Bone scanning is more sensitive than plain radiography and indicated when a stress or acute fracture is suspected and radiographs are negative.
- Base of fifth metatarsal fractures and Jones fractures can mostly be treated in non-weight bearing plaster of Paris.
- Shaft fractures of the metatarsals should be assessed as any other fracture in terms of displacement and angulation. Normally 10° of deviation in the dorsal/plantar plane or 3–4mm of translation in any plane requires active correction; manipulation or gravitational traction.

Section Three:

Practical procedures

CHAPTER 27

Aspiration of the elbow joint

Sam Oussedik and Fares Haddad

Indications

Indications for aspiration and injection of the elbow joint include:

- Osteoarthritis.
- Rheumatoid arthritis.
- Crystal arthropathies.
- Septic arthritis.
- Radial head fractures.

The technique described can be used for any of the above conditions. Aspiration of the elbow joint following radial head fracture will form the focus of this chapter.

Fractures to the radial head typically follow a fall onto the outstretched hand. Patients present with limited, painful elbow motion in both flexion/extension and pronation/supination. Tenderness may be elicited on palpation of the radial head. A haemarthrosis is present – this is seen as the 'fat pad' sign on X-ray. Diagnosis is confirmed by two-plane radiography (*Figures 27.1a* and *b*).

Aspiration serves three functions in radial head fractures:

- Confirms diagnosis: the aspirate contains blood and fat globules.
- Provides analgesia: relieves the capsular distension caused by haemarthrosis and by instilling a local anaesthetic agent.
- Allows examination of range of motion under local anaesthesia to assess for the presence of a mechanical block.

Planning

Having selected the patient with a suspected or radiologically proven radial head fracture, the clinician must prepare the necessary equipment to carry out the aspiration and infiltration of local anaesthetic. A collar and cuff must also be prepared to hold the arm following the procedure.

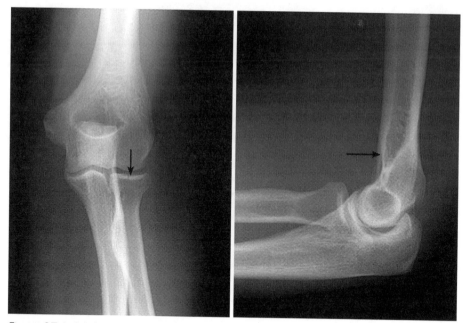

Figure 27.1. (a) Anteroposterior radiograph of elbow showing undisplaced radial head fracture (arrow). (b) Lateral radiograph of elbow showing fat pad sign (arrow).

Technique

Equipment

The following equipment is required:

- Sterile gloves.
- Skin preparation: iodine based or chlorhexidine.
- Sterile gauze.
- 5ml syringe.
- 22 gauge needle (blue).
- 2.5ml of 2% lidocaine (lignocaine) and 0.5% marcain in a labelled syringe.
- Adhesive dressing.

Procedure

The patient is positioned sitting on a couch with the arm resting on a side table. The elbow is placed in 45° of flexion. A sterile field is prepared by cleansing the skin over the lateral aspect of the elbow using the skin preparation and sterile gauze. The elbow joint is approached laterally, avoiding the ulnar nerve. The landmarks to palpate are illustrated in *Figure 27.2*. The needle is

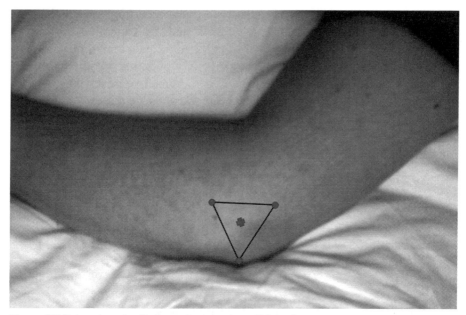

Figure 27.2. Landmarks for lateral aspiration of the elbow joint.

mounted onto the empty 5ml syringe. The site for insertion of the needle is the centre of a triangle formed by the radial head, the lateral epicondyle and the tip of the olecranon. The needle is then advanced in the direction of the medial epicondyle.

The syringe is aspirated as the needle is advanced. If a haemarthrosis is present, entry to the joint capsule is signalled by the aspiration of blood. The joint is aspirated until dry. The syringe is then disengaged from the needle, taking care not to dislodge the tip from the joint. The aspirate may then be decanted into a sterile container. Examination of the fluid once it has been allowed to settle may demonstrate fat globules. The fluid can then be sent for further microbiological or biochemical analysis as required.

The 2.5ml syringe is then mounted onto the needle which has remained within the elbow joint. The lidocaine and marcain can be infiltrated into the joint. The needle is finally withdrawn and an adhesive sterile dressing placed over the injection site.

A theoretical risk of introducing infection to the joint exists, and therefore all precautions must be taken to avoid this by the use of a meticulous aseptic technique.

Post-procedure

Following aspiration of the elbow and injection of the local anaesthetic, the elbow can be examined for the presence of a mechanical block to flexion or rotation. In the case of displaced radial head fractures, a fragment can become interposed between the radial head remnant and the capitellum, causing a mechanical block to movement. Having abolished the pain inhibition caused by the haemarthrosis, any residual loss of range of motion may be the result of a mechanical block. This may be an indication for operative treatment.

Aspiration of the elbow in radial head fractures increases the speed of recovery, as a full range of motion is restored more quickly and patients are more able to comply with physiotherapy (Holdsworth *et al*, 1987; Dooley and Angus, 1991).

Key points

■ Aspiration of radial head fracture haematoma and injection of local anaesthetic allows assessment for mechanical block to flexion.

■ The needle is introduced at a point at the centre of a triangle formed by the lateral epicondyle of the humerus, the tip of the olecranon and the lateral aspect of the radial head.

■ Aspiration of the elbow following radial head fracture improves the rate of recovery.

References

Dooley JF, Angus PD (1991) The importance of elbow aspiration when treating radial head fractures. *Arch Emerg Med* **8**(2): 117–21

Holdsworth BJ, Clement DA, Rothwell PN (1987) Fractures of the radial head – the benefit of aspiration: a prospective controlled trial. *Injury* **18**(1): 44–7

CHAPTER 28

Reduction of the dislocated shoulder

Sam Oussedik and Fares Haddad

Indications

The glenohumeral joint is the most commonly dislocated major joint of the body. Patients presenting with a suspected dislocation should be fully assessed as previously described. Of clinical importance are the distal neurovascular status, including axillary nerve function as examined through 'regimental patch' sensation, and the type of dislocation, anterior, posterior or inferior (luxatio erecta). The protocols described below apply to the reduction of the commonest type of injury, anterior dislocation. Posterior and inferior dislocations warrant discussion with the on-call orthopaedic team.

Anterior glenohumeral dislocation is diagnosed clinically, through the loss of normal shoulder contour, and the palpable anterior humeral head. Three plane X-rays including anteroposterior (AP), axillary and scapula Y views confirm the diagnosis (*Figure 28.1*). The radiographs may also highlight associated injuries, such as humeral neck injuries in the elderly, greater tuberosity fractures or Hill–Sachs lesions (indentations to the humeral head resulting from dislocation). The patient's general condition should also be documented as part of a full history and examination. This may help with decisions regarding appropriate anaesthesia.

Planning

Having confirmed the diagnosis and documented the neurovascular status of the arm, consideration must be given to both the type of anaesthesia, if any, to be used, and the method of reduction. A sling should be prepared to immobilise the arm following reduction. This should preferably hold the arm in adduction and internal rotation, but a broad arm sling may be used.

Anaesthetic options

Three types of anaesthesia are available in the accident and emergency department. These are:

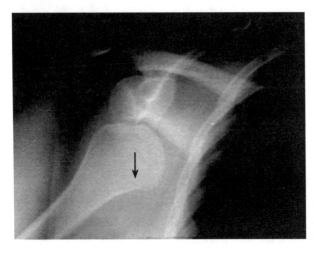

Figure 28.1. Anteroposterior view of anterior planohumeral dislocation.

- no anaesthesia (analgesia alone)
- local anaesthesia
- sedation and analgesia.

No anaesthesia

The main difficulty to overcome in reducing the dislocated shoulder is the spasm present in the shoulder musculature. However, in cases of recurrent dislocation of a pathologically lax shoulder, or in the elderly with weak musculature, this may be overcome without resorting to specific anaesthetic measures. This does not mean that the patient should not receive adequate analgesia, however, and this should be provided in all cases.

Local anaesthesia

Equipment
Equipment includes:

- 20ml syringe
- 20ml of 1% lidocaine (lignocaine) (maximum dose 4mg/kg)
- 20 gauge needle
- skin preparation (iodine based or chlorhexidine)
- sterile gauze
- dressing.

Technique
The patient sits at a comfortable angle on a trolley. A sterile field is prepared around the shoulder, using the skin preparation and sterile gauze. The

dislocated humeral head results in a depression just below the acromial edge, known as the lateral sulcus sign. The site for injection of the lidocaine is 2cm below the lateral or posterolateral acromial edge. The tip of the needle is directed towards the empty glenoid cavity. The syringe is aspirated to ensure the needle does not lie intravascularly. A small volume of lidocaine is injected at first, and a note is made of the resistance to injection. If correctly positioned, there should be minimal resistance. If resistance is encountered then the needle should be repositioned, and resistance reassessed. Once correctly positioned, the rest of the lidocaine is injected. The patient is allowed to rest for 5 minutes until the local anaesthetic has taken effect. Reduction can then be attempted.

Sedation and analgesia

Equipment
Equipment includes:

- 18 or 20 gauge intravenous (IV) cannula
- 5mg of morphine in labelled syringe
- 10mg of midazolam in labelled syringe
- oxygen and mask
- 20ml of 0.9% saline in labelled syringe
- pulse oximeter
- electrocardiogram (ECG) monitoring
- defibrillator, advanced life support equipment and drugs.

Technique
The patient should be starved. Informed written consent is obtained. Baseline observations are recorded. ECG and pulse oximeter monitoring are established. Oxygen is provided. The cannula is inserted into the contralateral arm and 5mg of morphine is given by slow intravenous injection. Five minutes are allowed to pass for the morphine to take effect. The midazolam is then given by slow intravenous injection. An initial dose of 1.5mg is provided. Further boluses are then titrated to effect, allowing 1–2 minutes between injections. Saline flushes are administered between doses. Adequate sedation is achieved once the eyelids begin to droop. Further doses can be administered once manipulation has been attempted if sedation is inadequate. The total dose of midazolam necessary is usually 3.5–7.5mg; in the elderly 3.5mg should be the maximum dose provided. Monitoring is continued throughout the recovery period, and the patient is not discharged until he/she is able to eat and drink. The patient must be accompanied home.

Greater muscular relaxation may be achieved through sedation and analgesia. However, intra-articular lidocaine has the advantage of being quicker and simpler to apply, requiring less observation following the procedure and allowing earlier discharge. As with any invasive technique, a theoretical risk of introducing infection exists, and all precautions must be taken to avoid this.

Techniques for reduction

A number of techniques are described for the reduction of anterior glenohumeral dislocation. Outlined below are those in common usage. Selection should depend on patient factors such as age and fragility of bones, injury factors such as the presence of associated fractures, and operator experience and preference. No prospective randomised controlled trial exists comparing the various techniques.

Traction–countertraction

This is perhaps the simplest technique. An assistant is necessary to provide the countertraction. The patient is positioned supine. The operator takes hold of the patient's forearm which is held in a neutral position with the elbow extended. The assistant loops a pillow case or sheet around the axilla and applies countertraction while the operator applies traction to the forearm. This is held for up to 5 minutes of steady traction. Success is signalled by an audible 'clunk' as the humeral head reduces. It is important to apply a steady force to the arm and to avoid any sudden jerks.

The Hippocratic technique

This is a variation on the traction–countertraction technique. It has the advantage of being carried out by a single operator, but is less elegant. The assistant's countertraction is replaced by the operator's foot being placed in the axilla. Steady traction and countertraction is then applied in a similar manner to that described above.

The external rotation technique

The external rotation technique (Leidelmeyer, 1977) is also sometimes called the Kocher method. The patient is positioned in a supine position. The elbow is flexed and held at a 90° angle. The operator's other hand holds the wrist and applies longitudinal traction. Once traction has been established over a period of several minutes to allow relaxation of the shoulder musculature, the arm is very slowly externally rotated. This is halted every few degrees to allow further relaxation. The arm is simultaneously slowly adducted across the chest.

Reduction is achieved following 5 minutes of this procedure, once the arm has reached the coronal plane and is at right angles to the body. Reduction may also be effected if the forearm is internally rotated once full external rotation and adduction has been achieved.

Stimson's technique

The patient is positioned in the prone position, with the affected arm hanging vertically over the edge of the couch. In this position, the operator can either apply weights to the forearm, beginning with 5lb and increasing to 15lb as necessary, or manually apply downward pressure. In either case, 15–20 minutes of pressure are necessary to effect reduction. Traction on the arm in this position allows the scapula to rock anteriorly, increasing the anteversion of the glenoid cavity and facilitating reduction.

The Milch technique

This technique was developed by Milch (1938). The patient is positioned in the supine position. The operator places one hand on the patient's shoulder with the thumb supporting the dislocated humeral head. The operator's other hand then takes hold of the patient's forearm and gently abducts it until it comes to lie above the patient's head. The humeral head is fixed in position such that it is rotated in its dislocated position. This allows the force exerted by the shoulder musculature to be eliminated, and the humeral head is then gently pushed back into position.

Reduction in elderly patients

In the elderly population with osteopenic bones, a method which avoids forceful rotation should be selected because of the potential risk of iatrogenic humeral fracture. The traction–countertraction technique can be safely used in this population.

Reduction in younger patients

Reduction may be unsuccessful in the younger population where muscular spasm is difficult to overcome. Associated greater tuberosity fracture may also mechanically block reduction. In such cases, reduction under general anaesthesia or open reduction should be considered.

Post-reduction

Following successful reduction, three plane radiographs should be repeated to both document reduction and reassess the presence of associated injuries. The distal neurovascular status is also reassessed and documented. The patient is discharged in an appropriate sling. Follow-up should be arranged according to local protocols.

Key points

- Glenohumeral dislocation is commonly seen in emergency departments.
- A number of anaesthetic options are available, choice often depending on local protocols and clinician preference.
- Care should be taken when making a choice of reduction technique in order to avoid iatrogenic injury.

References

Leidelmeyer R (1977) Reduced! A shoulder subtly and painlessly. *J Emerg Med* **9**: 233

Milch H (1938) Treatment of dislocation of the shoulder. *Surgery* **3**: 732–40

CHAPTER 29

Joint and soft tissue aspiration and injection

Rahul Patel and Fares Haddad

Introduction

The indications for joint or soft tissue aspiration and injection fall into two categories: diagnostic and therapeutic. A common diagnostic indication for placing a needle in a joint is the aspiration of synovial fluid for evaluation. Synovial fluid evaluation can differentiate among various joint disease aetiologies including infection, inflammation, and trauma. A second diagnostic indication involves the injection of a local anaesthetic to confirm the presumptive diagnosis through symptom relief of the affected body part. Therapeutic indications for joint or soft tissue aspiration and injection include decreased mobility and pain, and the injection of medication as a therapeutic adjunct to other forms of treatment.

Therapeutic injection with corticosteroids should always be viewed as adjuvant therapy. The improper or indiscriminate use of corticosteroids is likely to have a bad outcome. These injections should never be undertaken without diagnostic definition and a specific treatment plan in place.

Timing

Appropriate timing can minimise complications and allow a clear diagnosis or therapeutic response. For diagnostic injections, the procedure should be performed when acute or chronic symptoms are present, when the diagnosis is unclear or needs to be confirmed, when consideration has been given to other diagnostic modalities, and when septic arthritis has been ruled out (by aspiration and fluid analysis). For therapeutic injections, the procedure should be performed when acute or chronic symptoms are present, after the diagnosis and therapeutic plan have been made, and after consideration has been given to obtaining radiographs. Therapeutic injection should be performed only with or after the initiation of other therapeutic modalities (eg. physiotherapy).

Table 29.1. Contraindications to injection and aspiration

Contraindications to intra-articular or soft tissue injection	Contraindications to joint or or tissue needle aspiration
Adjacent osteomyelitis	Bacteraemia
Bacteraemia	Overlying infection in the soft tissues
Haemarthrosis	Severe coagulopathy
Impending (scheduled within days)	Severe overlying dermatitis
joint replacement surgery	Clinician unfamiliar with anatomy
Septic arthritis	of or approach to the joint
Osteochondral fracture	
Periarticular cellulitis	
Uncontrolled bleeding disorder or coagulopathy	

Complications

A number of potential complications can arise from the use of joint and soft tissue procedures. Local infection is always possible, but it can be avoided by following the proper technique. Joint injections should always be performed using sterile procedure to prevent iatrogenic septic arthritis. Local reactions at the injection site may include swelling, tenderness, and warmth, all of which may develop a few hours after injection and can last up to two days. A post-injection steroid flare, thought to be a crystal-induced synovitis caused by preservatives in the injectable suspension, may occur within the first 24–36 hours after injection. This is self-limited and responds to application of ice packs for no longer than 15-minute intervals.

Soft tissue (fat) atrophy and local depigmentation are possible with any steroid injection into soft tissue, particularly at superficial sites (eg. lateral epicondyle). Periarticular calcifications are described in the literature, but they are rare. Tendon rupture can be avoided by not injecting directly into the tendon itself.

Systemic effects are possible (especially after triamcinolone acetonide injection or injection into a vein or artery), and patients should always be acutely monitored for reactions. Alterations in taste have been reported for 1–2 days after steroid injection. Hyperglycaemia is possible in patients who have diabetes.

To avoid direct needle injury to articular cartilage or local nerves, attention should be paid to anatomic landmarks and depth of injection. Other rare, but possible, complications include perilymphatic depigmentation, steroid arthropathy, adrenal suppression, and abnormal uterine bleeding.

Contraindications to joint injection and aspiration are shown in *Table 29.1*.

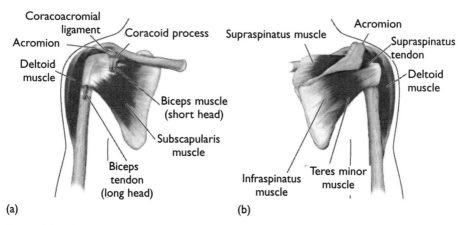

Figure 29.1. Anatomy of the shoulder and rotator cuff, showing (a) anterior and (b) posterior views.

Subacromial space injection

Subacromial space injection is used for several reasons. The first is for determining whether shoulder pain is the result of rotator cuff inflammation (tendinitis) or rotator cuff disruption (tear). Subacromial injection of anaesthetic takes just minutes and can eliminate the need for ultrasound or magnetic resonance imaging (MRI). Pain can inhibit muscle contraction, mimicking weakness secondary to a tear. Injection of the subacromial space relieves the pain. If strength returns after injection, the cause of the pain is more likely to be inflammation than disruption, and should be treated with aggressive physiotherapy. If strength does not return, the cause may be a tear. At this point, the patient may need surgical evaluation, including an MRI.

A second common reason for the procedure is to distinguish acromioclavicular (AC) joint pain from subacromial pain. This involves a two-step sequence of injection of the AC joint with 1.0–1.5ml of anaesthetic, followed by injection of the subacromial space, if necessary. The solution for injection of the AC joint can contain all short-acting anaesthetic, equal parts short- and long-acting anaesthetic, or 5–10mg steroid with anaesthetic.

Subacromial space injection can also be used for injection of corticosteroid to reduce inflammation and to achieve long-term pain relief for tendinitis and bursitis (impingement syndrome). This method for 'curing' tendinitis has not been documented in clinical studies, but has resulted in short- and long-term pain relief. Corticosteroid is not required for diagnostic injections, but many clinicians include it with the hope of longer pain relief.

A good knowledge of anatomy is vital, as for any attempted injection of a joint or soft tissue area (*Figure 29.1*).

The entry point for injection should be identified and marked with an impression from a thumbnail, a needle cap, or an indelible ink pen. The risk of infection at the site should be minimised. Prepare the area with an alcohol or povidone-iodine (Betadine) wipe. For all intra-articular injections, sterile technique should be used.

Although there are several entry points for shoulder injections, the posterior subacromial approach is the easiest. Furthermore, by angling the needle to the underside of the acromion, the physician can easily verify that the needle is properly positioned and, since the humeral head lies more anteriorly, there is no danger of hitting it.

Method

The patient should sit with the arms resting on the lap. Clothing should be removed so that a wide area posteriorly is exposed.

The posterior tip and inferior border of the acromion should be palpated. The thumb is placed on the inferior border and the index finger of the same hand on the coracoid process anteriorly. The entry point, 1–2cm medial to the tip of the acromion, under the thumb palpating the inferior border is marked.

A wide area of skin is cleaned with povidone-iodine solution. Local anaesthetic infiltration of skin is usually unnecessary but may be used in the anxious patient.

A separate syringe containing local anaesthetic with or without steroid is prepared and well mixed. Ideally a 20 gauge needle is used for injection.

Place the thumb and index finger of the non-injecting hand on the inferior border of the acromion and coracoid process; the direction between the two digits indicates the aim and direction of the needle. The needle is inserted through the entry point and directed towards the coracoid process; this angle is important because a needle angled medial to the coracoid process in the horizontal plane will enter the glenoid space; a give may be felt as the needle passes into the subacromial space.

Entry into the subacromial space is usually simple, but if the acromion or head of the humerus is encountered during joint entry, back the needle off and advance slowly with the redirected needle. An unexpected increase in resistance may indicate entry into ligament or the supraspinatus tendon.

The needle should be inserted to nearly its full length. Before injecting into the space, aspirate to ensure there is no return of blood. If there is unexpected flow resistance to the injection, withdraw the needle slightly to see if the flow resistance decreases.

Following withdrawal of the needle, dress the puncture wound with antibiotic ointment and an adhesive sterile dressing.

Calcific tendinitis

Calcific tendinitis of the shoulder causes pain that is not activity dependent and often severe. Its cause is uncertain and calcium deposits can be asymptomatic, so diagnosis is primarily by history and examination in conjunction with X-rays. Tenderness over the greater tuberosity generally differentiates calcific tendinitis from other conditions. For subacute and acute forms, needling (use of a hypodermic needle to disrupt deposits) followed by corticosteroid injection into the subacromial space can be diagnostic and therapeutic. The needling technique is different from that of subacromial space injection and is the most effective method of pain relief for this.

Subacute calcific tendinitis can be treated with oral non-steroidal anti-inflammatory medication and rest, but if signs and X-rays confirm calcific tendinitis, early needling and injection of the area is appropriate because the response is often diagnostic. Needling is believed to allow the encapsulated, pressurised deposit to decompress and permit vascular contact for calcium resorption and neovascularisation.

The midpoint of the acromion laterally is marked, having palpated anterior and posterior borders. The skin is prepared as described above and may be infiltrated with local anaesthetic. Using a syringe and a 20 gauge needle loaded with local anaesthetic and steroid, the needle is directed perpendicular to the surface of the skin. The needle will pass through the deltoid muscle into the firm tissue of the rotator cuff. If further anaesthesia is necessary for patient comfort, withdraw the needle from the cuff tissue just until it is free of resistance, and inject a small amount of the mixture. Then make passes with the needle into the rotator cuff to locate the calcium deposit, which will have a gritty texture. Insert the needle into the deposit four or five times to break it up, taking care not to inject any of the solution into the tendon. Withdraw the needle just until it clears the rotator cuff tissue and redirect it into the subacromial space. Then inject the mixture of lignocaine and corticosteroid into the subacromial bursa.

For both techniques, the patient must be advised to avoid strenuous activity of the affected area for several days after injection because of the small risk of local tissue tears secondary to temporarily high concentrations of steroid. This risk lessens as the steroid dissipates. Patients should look for signs of infection including erythema, warmth, or swelling at the injection site, or systemic signs including fever and chills. The patient should keep the injection site clean and may bathe.

Key points

- The indications for joint or soft tissue aspiration are diagnostic or therapeutic.
- Injection of corticosteroid should be part of a treatment plan for a specific diagnosis.
- Surface anatomical knowledge is an absolute prerequisite.

CHAPTER 30

Principles of plaster application

Claire Young and Fares Haddad

Introduction

The principle of management of any fracture is to reduce the fracture, immobilise until bony union is achieved and then rehabilitate the patient. There are various methods of fracture immobilisation varying from simple custom-made splints or plaster application for non-operative methods to various different operative techniques.

A fracture means loss of continuity and mechanical integrity of a bone. The bone ends bleed forming a fracture haematoma and this sets up a cascade of events that stimulates callus formation which is then replaced by bone through endochondral ossification, leading to fracture union and bone remodelling. Some movement is useful in stimulating this process; however, excessive motion is detrimental to these events and will lead to fracture non-union.

Splint immobilisation of fractures has been used for hundreds of years but gypsum was first used by Antonius Mathijsen in 1854. He was a Flemish military surgeon and used gypsum impregnated dressings to splint battlefield injuries.

Cast immobilisation can be divided into two groups. Holding casts are used to splint undisplaced stable fractures. Moulding casts use external contours to hold the fracture reduction.

Displaced or angulated fractures require fracture reduction to obtain satisfactory bony alignment. Once reduced the fracture requires adequate support to maintain the reduced position and overcome the deforming forces on the fracture fragments.

Longitudinal traction of the involved limb will overcome the muscle spasm restoring bone length and disimpacting the fracture. This can be achieved either by simple manual traction in line of the limb or application of Chinese finger traps to the digits for disimpaction of distal radius fractures. The latter relies on gradual traction to lead to muscle fatigue and overcome the spasm.

An understanding of the mechanism of injury sustained will aid in reduction of the fracture as reversing this mechanism should allow for restoring the anatomical bony alignment. For example, a fracture of the distal radius from a fall on the outstretched hand results from supination and dorsal angulation of

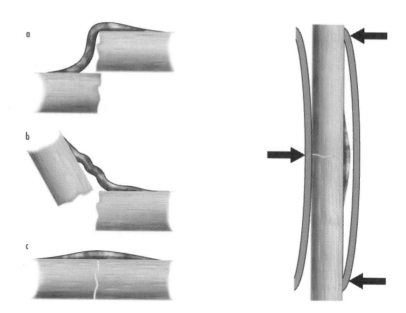

Figure 30.1. (left) Diagrammatic representation of intact soft tissue hinge. (a) Intact soft tissue hinge preventing fracture reduction. (b) Relaxation of soft tissue hinge allows bone ends to be reduced. (c) Once reduced soft tissue hinge helps maintain fracture reduction. Figure 30.2. (right) Principle of three-point moulding.

the distal fragments. To reduce this fracture following longitudinal traction of the forearm the wrist requires pronation and flexion to restore the anatomical alignment of the distal radius.

Frequently following fractures there is an intact periosteal soft tissue hinge. This can sometimes impede bony reduction. In this situation the soft tissue hinge needs to be relaxed by increasing the deformity before applying the longitudinal traction in order overcome this block to reduction. Once the fracture has been reduced this hinge of soft tissue aids in maintaining fracture reduction (*Figure 30.1*).

Plasters can be applied either as temporary splints or as definitive circumferential casts. Following an acute injury and fracture reduction it is often unwise to place the injured limb in a circumferential cast, as the limb will tend to swell. Circumferential casts may risk the development of compartment syndrome and in these cases it is often safer to apply a moulded plaster backslab which will adequately hold the fracture immobilised but still allow for swelling of the limb. The cast can then be completed or changed to a circumferential cast at a week once the initial acute swelling has subsided.

Plaster immobilisation of fractures should follow a few basic principles. In order to maintain fracture reduction three-point moulding should be

Table 30.1. Suggested plaster sizes for different anatomical sites

Anatomical region	Plaster width
Thigh	15cm
Leg	10cm
Upper limb	6cm

used (*Figure 30.2*). This produces tension on the side of the fracture with an intact soft tissue hinge. The initial deformity should be overcorrected. Successful moulding should result in a curved cast to immobilise a straight bone (Charnley, 1999). In fractures involving rotational deforming forces the joint above and below the fracture should be immobilised in the early phase to prevent limb rotation.

Cast application

Tubular stockinette is applied to the limb. Circumferential wadding is then applied the length of the limb to be immobilised. Too much tension should be avoided in the wadding to prevent a tourniquet affect. The wadding should be applied evenly and overlap approximately 50% of its width for each turn. Too much padding reduces the effectiveness of the cast, sufficient needs to be applied to adequately protect bony prominences (eg. malleoli) from pressure effects.

A plaster roll of appropriate width (*Table 30.1*) is selected. It should be unrolled approximately 5cm and immersed in lukewarm water, keeping hold of the roll and the end, until all the air bubbles have dispersed. The plaster should be applied to the limb in the same direction as the wadding overlapping each turn by approximately 50% the width of the roll (*Figure 30.3*). The aim is to achieve a plaster of even thickness throughout its length. The plaster should be smoothed using the thenar eminences, and moulded with a three-point technique appropriately as it sets. The ends of the plaster can be trimmed back to the appropriate length.

Lower limb backslabs require careful application as they necessitate not only a plaster slab on the posterior aspect of the limb but also a U slab wound from medial to lateral over the heel to give varus/valgus and rotational stability. Following cotton wadding being wound around the limb from the metatarsal heads for the appropriate length of the leg to be immobilised the wetted U slab plaster is applied first (*Figure 30.4*). The wetted posterior slab is then applied (if the plaster is applied in this order then the U slab helps to hold the posterior slab while the securing bandage is wound over the top. By commencing the

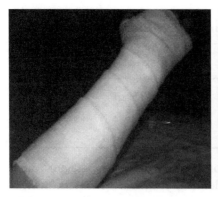
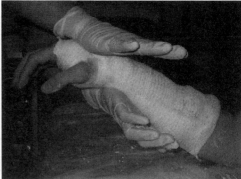

Figure 30.3. Application of wadding and moulding of forearm cast.

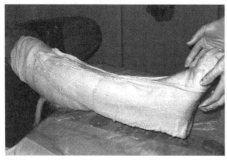
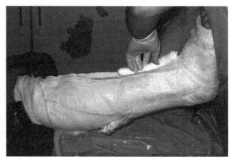

Figure 30.4. Application of below-knee U slab.

Figure 30.5. Completion of backslab by dorsiflexion of ankle and applying securing bandage from distal to proximal.

securing bandaging at the metatarsal heads the posterior slab can be secured in place appropriately and the foot brought up to a neutral position at the ankle by gentle pressure on the sole of the foot (*Figure 30.5*).

Non-operative treatment of fractures with cast immobilisation is labour intensive. Patients require frequent evaluation (both clinical and radiological) in the early phase of their treatment, as this is the period of greatest fracture instability while early callus is formed to help stabilise the fracture. As the swelling from the initial injury subsides the cast no longer fits snugly around the limb. This allows space for the deforming forces to displace the fracture fragments.

Clinical bony union frequently precedes radiological fracture union and treatment of a patient in a cast relies on careful regular evaluation to determine bony union. If the cast is left in situ until radiological union is achieved then the fracture has been overtreated and the adjacent joints will have become excessively stiff, and the patient's rehabilitation delayed.

Key points

- Cast immobilisation can provide temporary stabilisation or definitive treatment of fractures.
- Plaster immobilisation of fractures relies on good three-point fixation to maintain fracture reduction.
- In general principles the joint above and below the fracture should be immobilised by the plaster.
- Definitive treatment of fractures by plaster immobilisation requires careful, regular clinical and radiological assessments of the patient.

Reference

Charnley J (1999) *The Closed Treatment of Common Fractures.* The Golden Jubilee Edition. Colt Books, Cambridge

CHAPTER 31

Spinal immobilisation

Benjamin Hudson, James Waller and Sam Oussedik

Introduction

The early recognition and correct management of spinal injuries is vital to avoid serious, irreversible long-term consequences. In the 1970s the American College of Surgeons (ACS) devised the Advanced Trauma Life Support (ATLS) course. This was designed to give any doctor the basic knowledge to stabilise any trauma patient in a systematic fashion. These guidelines are still widely accepted as the gold standard for the assessment and initial management of trauma patients throughout the world.

One of the many issues addressed by the ACS was that of spinal immobilisation. Following blunt trauma, vertebral column injury is common. It should therefore be assumed that spinal cord injury has occurred until proven otherwise. Without correct immobilisation of the spine, an unstable vertebral column can cause or exacerbate a spinal cord injury. Excessive manipulation of the spine during transfer, assessment and management of a trauma patient means that medical intervention can lead to iatrogenic injury.

Spinal injury

In most cases trauma patients will arrive in the accident and emergency department already immobilised by the paramedic team. However, the patient still needs to be transferred safely from the ambulance to the hospital examining table.

Once the spine is immobilised appropriately, examination and imaging of the spine can be deferred while other, more immediately life-threatening problems are treated. The patient should remain immobilised until spinal injury is excluded.

A sound knowledge of the natural anatomical position and neuroanatomy of the spine is vital when applying immobilisation. Failure to immobilise the spine correctly can lead to further injury.

Immobilisation

Spinal immobilisation should be applied in such a way as to keep the patient in completely neutral alignment. There should be no rotation, forward or lateral flexion, or extension of any part of the spine. This is most important in the cervical region, where the majority of spinal column injuries occur.

The use of a cervical collar, long spinal board and bolstering devices can limit neck movements by up to 95%. The widely used semi-rigid cervical collar can be placed, after correct sizing, around the neck with minimal manipulation of the patient. These are designed to limit cervical motion to 11° in all planes. They do not provide sufficient immobilisation on their own, however.

The long spinal board provides an effective spinal splint. The spinal board is also used to transfer the patient between trolleys and surfaces.

Lastly a variety of bolstering devices and straps keep the patient in neutral alignment on the board or table. The patient's head and neck can be bolstered with specifically designed head blocks placed either side of the head above the shoulders. Makeshift bolsters can be fashioned from saline bags or sandbags. Straps are then used to secure the patient to the spinal board at the forehead, neck, chest, pelvis and ankles.

The log roll

The most difficult and potentially dangerous element of immobilisation is the log roll. This technique is used to transfer the patient between surfaces without compromising the integrity of the spine. The initial log roll will be to move the patient from the scene to the ambulance spinal board, and then from the ambulance long board to the hospital table. It is important that the patient is removed quickly from the long spinal board to a firm, padded hospital examination table. During this final transfer, it is a good opportunity to expose and examine the back, thereby omitting another unnecessary movement.

An effective, safe log roll requires at least four trained members of the trauma team (*see Figures 6.4–6.7, Chapter 6*). The first person stands at the head of the table immobilising and maintaining neutral alignment of the cervical spine. This is done by placing one hand on each shoulder and then using the forearms to bolster the patient's head between them. This minimises cervical motion as much as possible.

The second person's responsibility is to control the torso and arms, thereby stabilising the thoracolumbar spine. The arms are straightened and placed by the patient's side, palms in, and the clinician holds the shoulder furthest away and stabilises the wrist against the body.

The third member of the team stabilises the pelvis and the legs, by holding the hip furthest away, and the ankles, which are tied together. The team members controlling the body and legs will stand on the side of the table that the patient is to be rolled towards.

The last person is there to direct the procedure, and also to position or remove the spinal board. This person is also in a good position to inspect and palpate the patient's back during the log roll.

At the command of the person controlling the head and neck, the team in unison then rolls the patient towards the clinicians supporting the torso, pelvis and legs. The smallest degree of movement possible should be used to position or remove the spinal board and to inspect the back. The patient is then slowly and steadily lowered back down.

Complications

Spinal immobilisation is not without its risks and complications. The purpose of spinal boards is to provide a safe transferring mechanism. They are not designed for the patient to spend any lengthy amount of time on.

As soon as possible the patient should be transferred on to a firm, padded surface to prevent the formation of ulcers which can develop quickly. This may be compounded if there is a neurological deficit causing areas of anaesthesia.

For this reason it is recommended that the patient is removed from the spinal board in under 2 hours, and should also be regularly log-rolled once off the spinal board. Ulcers tend to form at the areas of most pressure, eg. sacrum, scapulae, heels and the occiput.

Other risks of spinal immobilisation include: difficult airway management; venous obstruction; difficult central venous access and care; decreased enteral feeding and increased risk of pulmonary aspiration.

Conclusions

At present in the UK there are no specific mandatory guidelines for managing the trauma patient. However the ACS's Advanced Trauma Life Support guidelines are widely used and endorsed by the British Orthopaedic Association and the Royal College of Surgeons.

There is a need for a nationally accepted protocol that should be constructed for accident and emergency, surgical and medical trainees early in their career.

The authors would like to thank Dr Heidi Artiss and Dr Sarah Thompson for their assistance with this chapter.

Key points

- Spinal cord injury in the trauma patient should be assumed to have occurred until proven otherwise.
- Effective spinal immobilisation is paramount to preventing or exacerbating cord injury.
- The log roll should be performed safely and steadily during transfer of patients and evaluation of the spine.
- Spinal immobilisation allows the clinician to manage other life-threatening problems, while maintaining the integrity of the spine.
- Spinal boards are recommended for transfer only, and patients should not be left on them for more than 2 hours.

Further reading

American College of Surgeons Committee on Trauma (1997) *Advanced Trauma Life Support for Doctors*. American College of Surgeons, Chicago

Bernhard M, Gries A, Kremer P, Martin-Villalba A, Bottiger BW (2005) Prehospital management of spinal cord injuries. *Der Anaesthetist* **54**: 357–76

Greaves I, Porter K, Burke D (1997) *Key Topics In Trauma*. Bios Scientific Publishers, Oxford

Hoff WS (2001) Evaluation and management of spinal cord injury. In: Sing RF, Reilly PM, eds. *Initial Management of Injuries*. BMJ Books, London: 35–43

Morris CG, McCoy EP, Lavery GG (2004) Spinal immobilisation for unconscious patients with multiple injuries. *Brit Med J* **329**: 495–9

Papadopoulos MC, Chakraborty A, Waldron G, Anthony Bell B (1999) Exacerbating cervical spine injury by applying a hard collar. *Brit Med J* **319**: 171–2

Santora TA, Kaplan LJ, Trooskin (2001) Evaluation of the Cervical Spine. In: Sing RF, Reilly PM, eds. *Initial Management of Injuries*. BMJ Books, London: 20–30

Swain A, Dove J, Baker H (2000) In: Driscoll P, Skinner D, Earlam R, eds. *ABC of Major Trauma*. 3rd edn. BMJ Books, London: 48–55

Tinkoff GH (2001) Evaluation of thoracolumbar vertebral column injury. In: Sing RF, Reilly PM, eds. *Initial Management of Injuries*. BMJ Books, London: 31–4

CHAPTER 32

Technique of knee joint aspiration

Rahul Patel and Fares Haddad

Anatomy and function

Knee joint aspiration and injection are performed to establish a diagnosis, relieve discomfort, drain off infected fluid, or instill medication.

The knee joint is the most common and the easiest joint for a clinician to aspirate. Because prompt treatment of a joint infection can preserve the joint integrity, any unexplained monoarthritis should be considered for arthrocentesis (*Table 32.1*). Arthrocentesis may also help distinguish the inflammatory arthropathies from the crystal arthritides or osteoarthritis. If a haemarthrosis is discovered after trauma, it can indicate the presence of a fracture (fat globules in the aspirate) or other anatomical disruption.

An effusion of the knee often produces detectable suprapatellar or parapatellar swelling. Large effusions can produce ballottement of the patella. Medial or lateral approaches to the knee can be selected; some advocate the medial approach when the effusion is small and the lateral approach with larger effusions. The lateral approach will be discussed here.

Method

- The knee generally is easiest to aspirate when the patient is supine and the knee is extended. A pillow may be placed under the knee for comfort and to relax the quadriceps muscle group.

Table I. Indications for knee joint aspiration

Crystal-induced arthropathy
Haemarthrosis
Suspected septic arthritis
Symptomatic relief from large effusion
Unexplained joint effusion
Unexplained monoarthritis

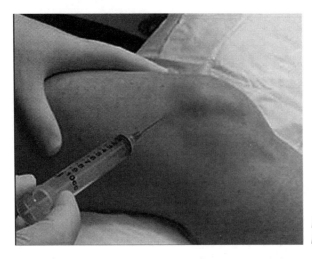

Figure 32.1. Superolateral knee joint aspiration.

- Identify the medial, lateral and superior borders of the patella. Check for overlying cellulitis or coexisting pathology in the joint or surrounding tissues.

- The superior lateral aspect of the patella is palpated. The skin is marked with a pen, one fingerbreadth above and one fingerbreadth lateral to this site (*Figure 32.1*). This location provides the most direct access to the synovium.

- A wide area of skin is cleaned with povidone-iodine solution. The skin and underlying dermis is infiltrated with local anaesthetic at the point where aspiration will take place so that a small bleb is raised. The needle may then be advanced to the subcutaneous tissues for further infiltration of local anaesthetic, with negative pressure applied to the syringe throughout to ensure no vasculature is injected.

- A fresh syringe (ideally 20ml) and large bore needle (18 gauge) is then used to aspirate the joint. The needle entry point is through the bleb, directed at a 45° angle distally and 45° into the knee, tilted below the patella, with negative pressure applied to the syringe throughout. The syringe should fill with fluid once the joint is entered. Using the non-dominant hand to compress the opposite side of the joint or the patella may aid in arthrocentesis.

- If the bore appears obstructed during the arthrocentesis, try rotating the needle or injecting some aspirate, attempting to clear the needle. If this fails, try reinserting the needle 1cm deeper or changing direction slightly. A give may be felt when the needle pierces the synovium.

- Aspirate as much fluid as possible, changing syringe when needed but keeping the needle in the joint.

- Following withdrawal of the needle, dress the iatrogenic puncture wound with an antibiotic ointment and appropriate adhesive sterile dressing.

Table 32.2. Contraindications to intra-articular injection

Adjacent osteomyelitis
Bacteraemia
Haemarthrosis
Impending (scheduled within days) joint replacement surgery
Septic arthritis
Osteochondral fracture
Periarticular cellulitis
Uncontrolled bleeding disorder or coagulopathy

Table 32.3. Contraindications to joint needle aspiration

Bacteraemia
Overlying infection in the soft tissues
Severe coagulopathy
Severe overlying dermatitis
Clinician unfamiliarity with anatomy of or approach to the joint

---

▪ Although rare, infection and haemarthrosis may complicate arthrocentesis. Application of a compression bandage may be indicated for haemarthrosis and large effusions.

Corticosteroid may be injected in the same manner. The use of local anaesthetic is not mandatory. There are many different techniques for aspirating or injecting the knee. These include medial, lateral and anterior approaches. Each has its own merit, but choice of approach is dependent on the clinician's preference. The lateral approach is most commonly used. For the medial approach, the needle enters the medial side of the knee under the middle of the patella (midpole) and is directed toward the opposite patellar midpole. In the anterior approach, the knee is flexed 60–90°, and the needle is inserted just medial or lateral to the patellar tendon and parallel to the tibial plateau. This technique is preferred by some for its ease of joint entry in advanced osteoarthritis. However, the anterior approach may incur greater risk of meniscal injury by the needle.

The indications, complications and pitfalls for knee arthrocentesis generally can be applied to other joints (*Tables 32.2* and *32.3*). Many of the principles of needle aspiration and injection also can be used for soft tissue disorders, such as bursitis or tendinitis.

All fluid is sent for investigation: microscopy, white cell count, gram stain,

Table 32.4. Typical condition-dependant characteristics of fluid aspirated

Type of fluid	Special features
Normal	Clear, colourless, viscous
Non-inflammatory	Clear, yellow, viscous
Inflammatory	Cloudy, yellow, watery. Glucose may be low
Septic	Purulent. Glucose very low

crystals, glucose and protein. Even a 'dry tap' can yield important and sufficient information and should not be discarded. The colour and appearance of the aspirate should be noted as this may direct initial suspicions (*Table 32.4*).

Experience is important for the proper performance of joint aspiration and injection procedures. Each joint has different anatomical landmarks, and novice clinicians may need to review a textbook for approaches to an unfamiliar joint. Although arthrocentesis is a simple technique with minimal risk, one should have assistance or supervision with the first attempt at any site.

Key points

- Knee joint aspiration and injection are performed to establish a diagnosis, relieve discomfort, drain off infected fluid, or instil medication.
- Medial or lateral approaches to the knee can be selected.
- In the lateral approach the skin is marked with a pen, one fingerbreadth above and one fingerbreadth lateral to this site.
- A wide area of skin is cleaned with povidone-iodine solution.
- The needle is directed at a 45° angle distally and 45° into the knee, tilted below the patella, with negative pressure applied to the syringe throughout.

CHAPTER 33

Manipulation and immobilisation of Colles' fractures

Sam Oussedik and Fares Haddad

Indications

Closed reduction and immobilisation within a plaster cast remains an acceptable treatment for the majority of distal radial fractures. In order to gain satisfactory results, it is important to select carefully which patients to manage in this manner.

In general, Colles' fractures, or those showing a combination of dorsal angulation, dorsal shift and radial shift following a fracture in osteopenic bone in patients over 50 years of age, are amenable to this type of management.

Patient factors to consider should include hand dominance, employment, functional demand and patient expectations. Injury factors to consider include displacement, articular involvement and comminution. Together these injury factors give an idea as to the relative stability of the injury, and therefore its tendency to redisplace following reduction. Choosing to manage non-operatively a dominant hand displaced comminuted intra-articular fracture in a young patient with moderate functional demand and high expectations is unlikely to meet with success.

Planning

Having selected the patient, a careful analysis of the injury pattern must be made before attempting reduction. Colles' fractures typically show a combination of dorsal angulation, dorsal shift and radial shift. In addition they also tend to be impacted. These are the deformities one must reverse in order to achieve as anatomical a reduction as possible. Before manipulation, one must prepare the equipment necessary to immobilise the fracture. This includes:

- Plaster of Paris, 6 or 8 inches wide, six sheets thick, with a section removed to accommodate the thumb.
- Lukewarm water in a bucket large enough to submerge the entire plaster of Paris bandage.

- Cotton wool bandage.
- 6-inch crepe bandage.
- Adhesive tape.

Anaesthesia

Having analysed the deformity, one must then decide on the type of anaesthesia to administer. Three main types are available in the accident and emergency department:

- Local anaesthesia with a haematoma block.
- Regional anaesthesia with a Bier's block.
- Sedation and analgesia.

The choice of anaesthesia may be dictated by local protocols. However, each has its own advantages and disadvantages.

Haematoma block

Equipment

- Sterile gloves.
- Betadine skin preparation.
- Sterile gauze swabs.
- 10ml syringe and 20 gauge needle.
- 10ml of sterile 1% lignocaine.
- Sterile cotton wool.

Technique

Informed written consent is obtained from the patient. Sterile gloves are donned. The forearm is cleaned with betadine-soaked gauze swabs. The syringe is filled with 10ml of 1% lignocaine. The dorsum of the wrist is gently palpated to locate the fracture.

The needle, mounted on the syringe, is then introduced percutaneously at 90° to the skin into the fracture site. Once the fracture site has been penetrated a flashback of blood will be seen in the barrel of the needle. Further aspiration should yield little more blood, differentiating the fracture site from a blood vessel. Once the operator is happy that the tip of the needle lies within the fracture site, 8–10ml of lignocaine is injected. The needle is then withdrawn, and the injection site covered with sterile cotton wool until bleeding has ceased. Adequate analgesia is achieved in 2–5 minutes, when gentle manipulation of the fracture site is relatively painless.

Bier's block

Equipment

- Bier's block machine (double-cuff tourniquet).
- 18 or 20 gauge intravenous cannula.
- 1% prilocaine – no other local anaesthetic should be used.
- 0.9% saline for dilution of prilocaine.
- Oxygen with mask.
- Pulse oximeter.
- Electrocardiographic (ECG) monitor.
- Defibrillator, advanced life support (ALS) equipment and drugs.

Technique

Contraindications to the use of a Bier's block include: hypertension (systolic blood pressure >200mmHg), sickle cell anaemia, children younger than 16 years of age, peripheral vascular disease, infection of the limb, fracture to the ipsilateral humerus, or compartment syndrome. When using a Bier's block, it is essential that two doctors are present: one to apply the block and monitor the patient, and another to manipulate the fracture. The patient should preferably be starved.

Informed written consent is obtained. The patient's baseline blood pressure and heart rate are recorded. The correct volume of prilocaine is prepared. The 1% prilocaine is diluted with an equal volume of 0.9% saline to produce a 0.5% solution. The dose of prilocaine is 3mg/kg, so for a 70kg patient this translates to 42ml. The gas pressure in the cylinders supplying the tourniquets is checked before starting.

The cannula is inserted into a suitable hand vein on the side to be anaesthetised. The tourniquets are applied to the upper arm on the affected side. The arm is elevated for 2 minutes to exsanguinate. The cuffs are then inflated to 100mmHg above systolic pressure. The prilocaine is then injected through the intravenous cannula. The patient should be monitored throughout the period of anaesthesia for evidence of toxicity. The signs to look out for are circumoral tingling, confusion, seizures, bradycardia and hypotension. The tourniquets should remain inflated for a minimum of 20 minutes following injection. The cannula is removed before discharge.

Sedation and analgesia

Equipment

- 18 or 20 gauge IV cannula.
- Morphine 5mg in labelled syringe.

- Midazolam 10mg in labelled syringe.
- Oxygen and mask.
- 20ml of 0.9% saline in labelled syringe.
- Pulse oximeter.
- ECG monitoring.
- Defibrillator, ALS equipment and drugs.

Technique

The patient should be starved. Informed written consent is obtained. Baseline observations are recorded. ECG and pulse oximeter monitoring are established. Oxygen is provided. The cannula is inserted into the contralateral arm. Morphine 5mg is given by slow intravenous injection. Five minutes are allowed to pass for the morphine to take effect. The midazolam is then given by slow intravenous injection. An initial dose of 1.5mg is provided. Further boluses are then titrated to effect, allowing 1–2 minutes to pass between injections. Saline flushes are administered between doses.

Adequate sedation is achieved once the eyelids begin to droop. Further doses can be administered once manipulation has been attempted if sedation is inadequate. The total dose of midazolam necessary is usually 3.5–7.5mg; in the elderly 3.5mg should be the maximum dose provided. Monitoring is continued throughout the recovery period, and the patient is not discharged until able to eat and drink. The patient must be accompanied home.

Advantages and disadvantages

A haematoma block is relatively quick and easy to carry out. However, the quality of analgesia is variable. No muscle relaxation is achieved, making manipulation more difficult. A theoretical risk of osteomyelitis also exists.

A Bier's block produces excellent analgesia and muscle relaxation, but involves specialised equipment and requires the presence of two doctors. There is also a risk of toxicity associated with the use of large volumes of prilocaine, especially if the cuffs fail or are let down too early.

Sedation and analgesia also produces good analgesia and muscle relaxation. The amnesic effects of midazolam are useful. However, there is a risk of producing too deep a sedation, leading to airway compromise. Careful monitoring is required throughout.

Kendall *et al* (1997) have shown that Bier's block is superior to haematoma block in terms of the reduction that can be achieved.

Manipulation

Figure 33.1 shows the typical radiographic appearances of a Colles' fracture.

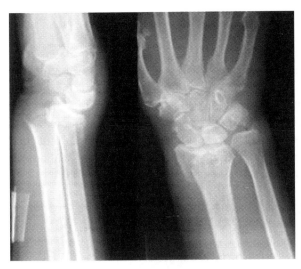

Figure 33.1. Typical radiological appearances of a Colles' fracture.

There is dorsal angulation of the distal fragment, together with dorsal and radial shift. These are the deformities that must be reversed in order to achieve an adequate reduction.

Having ensured adequate analgesia by any of the methods described above, and having prepared the necessary equipment for immobilisation in plaster, one can attempt to manipulate the fracture. Before manipulation, a stockingette bandage with a hole cut out for the thumb can be rolled up to the elbow.

Manipulation requires the use of an assistant to apply countertraction at the elbow. With the proximal forearm thus immobilised, one begins by applying in-line traction to the fracture. The dorsal deformity is then accentuated to aid with disimpaction. With traction maintained, the distal fragment is then flexed into a reduced position. Pressure is then applied to the radial aspect of the fragment with the heel of the hand to correct the radial shift. The fracture is now reduced, and is maintained in this position by flexing the wrist and pronating the forearm (Charnley, 1999).

The stockingette is now rolled down to cover the forearm, pulling the thumb through its hole. Cotton wool bandage is applied, paying particular care to providing adequate padding over possible pressure areas such as the ulna styloid. The stockingette and wool should cover the forearm from elbow to proximal interphalangeal joints of the fingers. The radial plaster of Paris slab is now applied. The ends of the stockingette and wool are rolled back to cover the ends of the plaster, and the crepe bandage is applied. Adhesive tape is used to secure the end of the crepe bandage. At this point moulding can be applied. Pressure is applied to the volar aspect of the wrist, followed by proximal pressure over the dorsum of the forearm and distal pressure over the dorsum of the proximal metacarpals. The wrist is immobilised in a position of slight flexion and ulnar deviation.

Post-manipulation

Once the patient has recovered from the anaesthetic, check radiographs must be obtained and the adequacy of reduction assessed. A broad arm sling can then be provided and the patient discharged with an appointment to return to fracture clinic for assessment 1 week later. At this appointment the injury will be X-rayed again to ensure that reduction has been maintained. If the reduction is maintained the backslab is completed to a full cast. In the event of reduction being lost, it may be necessary to remanipulate the fracture with or without the addition of percutaneous wires to increase stability.

Key points

- The majority of distal radial fractures are amenable to non-operative treatment.
- Patient selection is the key to ensuring success.
- A number of anaesthetic options are available, each with its own advantages and disadvantages.
- Careful follow-up is vital to ensure maintenance of reduction and recovery of function.

References

Charnley J (1999) *The Closed Treatment of Common Fractures*. Colt Books, Cambridge

Kendall JM, Allen P, Younge P, Meek SM, McCabe SE (1997) Haematoma block or Bier's block for Colles' fracture reduction in the accident and emergency department – which is best? *J Accid Emerg Med* **14**: 352–6

Index

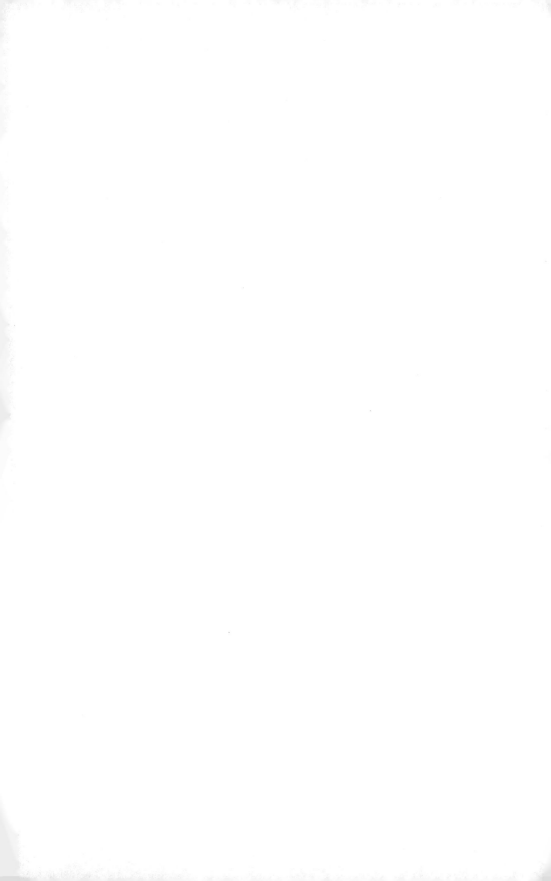